A Family Caregiver's Guide
to Planning and Decision Making
for the Elderly

James A. Wilkinson

Fairview Press
Minneapolis

Library of Congress Cataloging-in-Publication Data

Wilkinson, James A.
    A family caregiver's guide to planning and decision making for the elderly / James A. Wilkinson
       p.   cm.
    ISBN 1-57749-077-0 (alk. paper)
    1. Aged—Care—United States—Decision making.   2. Aged—Home care—United States.   3. Aging parents—Care—United States—Life skill guides.
    I. Title.
    HV1461.W518   1999
    362.6—DC21
                                     98-20198
                                         CIP

First Printing: January 1999
Printed in the United States of America
03 02 01 00 99   7 6 5 4 3 2 1

HCFA Nursing Home Checklist taken from the Health Care Financing Administration web site: http://www.hcfa.gov/medicare/nurshm4.htm.

Quotation reprinted with permission of Merck & Co. from *The Merck Manual of Geriatrics,* 2nd Edition, edited by William B. Abrams, Mark H. Beers, and Robert Berkow. Copyright 1995 by Merck & Co., Inc., Whitehouse Station, NJ, p 5.

Values History Form reprinted with the permission of the Center for Health, Law, and Ethics, Institute of Public Law, University of New Mexico School of Law.

Edited by: Rose Brandt and Stephanie Billecke
Interior: Dorie McClelland
Cover: *Cover Design by Laurie Duren*™

For a free current catalog of Fairview Press titles, please call toll-free 1-800-544-8207. Or visit our web site at www.Press.Fairview.org.

For my father, who, at ninety, keeps forcing me
to revise what elderly people can do; and for my wife,
with whom I genuinely hope to become an elderly person.

Contents

Acknowledgments

A number of people have been particularly helpful in the preparation of this book, but two stand out. Judy Hlafcsak, an attorney I have had the pleasure to work with as well as a good friend, was really the inspiration for this book. The original conception was hers, and she prodded me into writing it. While it started as a joint project, in the end she did not have time to be more than a reviewer.

The other person is my daughter, Katie. Her offer to look at a few chapters turned into several weeks of editing and questioning, and it has been a genuine pleasure working with her. Her insights and good humor were particularly helpful as I balanced finishing the book with my full-time career. Her talent with words is apparent. It's nice to know that her writing skills may exceed mine.

My wife, Susanne, has been very supportive of this project, especially in putting up with my inability to do other things while I was working on it.

Many others also contributed in ways large and small. In particular, I want to thank the people at Meritcare: Tom Konig, Jan Beresford, and especially Mike Cervo, whose insights were helpful in the financial sections. They kept the crises to a minimum and were generous in the time they gave me to work on this project. Also, Terrence Starz, M.D., and Peter Koenig, M.D., offered invaluable help with the medical sections.

Of course, I would also like to thank my editors at Fairview Press. Thanks to Lane Stiles, who took a chance on the book. And my special thanks to Stephanie Billecke, the editor with whom I have had the pleasure to work most closely. Not only has she put up with my comments and changes, she has been able to turn a rough manuscript into a useful and usable book.

How to Use This Book

This book is not designed to be read from front to back. Chapters are presented in no special order but are complete in themselves, with related information cross-referenced. For information on a specific topic, simply look through the table of contents or index and go to the correct page.

There are forms to fill out throughout the book. Some are simple, others are time-consuming. Some are easy to understand, others may require interpretation by a professional. In addition, some forms may not be relevant to your situation, while others will be useful over and over again. You may want to photocopy those forms you'll want to update regularly.

If you currently are in a situation that is gradually deteriorating, but not yet a crisis, focus on the sections that seem most important. By completing the forms in those sections, you will gain a deeper understanding of the elderly person's affairs. This will help you prepare for future decisions. Whenever possible, it's best to gather the information before a crisis occurs.

If, on the other hand, you are already in a crisis—especially a medical crisis—use the forms to help stabilize the situation before you try to tackle anything else. When an elderly person living alone is suddenly hospitalized, for example, many steps must be taken: friends and family must be contacted, bills must be paid, valuables must be stored for safekeeping, perishable food must be discarded, arrangements must be made for pet care, and newspapers and mail must be stopped. Once you have dealt with the immediate crisis, you can use the forms in this book to find out what to do next.

In addition to its extensive list of resources, this book covers many health, housing, legal, and financial issues. Remember, caring for the elderly is complex. Each situation is unique. You'll need to set up a filing system to maintain accurate records, such as notes of calls and conversations, and secure, accessible storage of forms and documents. The more organized you are, the easier it will be to quickly get help when help is needed.

This book is an organizational tool. It will not tell you how to convince your aging parent to turn in the car keys or how to handle your sister who refuses to agree to anything. Nor does it assume that you have nothing better to do than plan for every possible emergency. It is simply designed to help you collect and organize the information you (and any professionals you consult) will need to make informed decisions.

I have tried to make this book as complete, helpful, and accurate as possible. If you notice any missing or incorrect information, please notify me so I can correct it in future editions. You can contact me directly at wilkinso@bellatlantic.net or through the publisher.

Introduction

I wrote this book in response to the lack of useful information available to caregivers of the elderly. For several years, I had regularly fielded questions from desperate caregivers who wanted to know the answer to the question, "Now what do I do?" Sometimes I had the answers, and sometimes I didn't.

In my search for a book to recommend that would answer some of the routine questions caregivers ask, I found scattered information about aging, the elderly, and the caregiving process. What I did not find was a book that organized all this information into one comprehensible resource to help caregivers understand and prioritize options according to their unique situation.

A Family Caregiver's Guide to Planning and Decision Making for the Elderly is the result.

Organized to support the decision-making process, this book offers thorough, practical advice and assistance. It strives to do three things:

1. Provide detailed forms and checklists to address specific issues, such as organizing financial resources and important records, managing medications, and selecting a nursing home or home healthcare provider. Forms are included in this book to help you gather and organize essential information. You can make copies of these forms, or write your information directly in this book.

2. Prepare you for making key decisions, such as deciding if an elderly person should move, selecting an assisted-living facility, or completing a durable power of attorney.

3. Provide an extensive list of resources that offer detailed information. You will find plenty of information on topics specific to your caregiving situation in the resource chapter at the end of this book.

This book is written for the average caregiver. It assumes that you, the reader, are not a doctor, lawyer, pharmacist, social worker, or insurance agent well versed in issues affecting the elderly. Even if you are a professional in one of these fields, you may have limited expertise in the range of complex issues that face the elderly. A doctor may understand a patient's medical prognosis, for example, but he or she may have little knowledge of long-term care insurance, home safety, or Medicaid planning.

Though this book seeks to be a thorough, comprehensive guide, caregivers should always seek professional help when needed. And, the more knowledgeable that professional is about the elderly, the better.

For example, a gerontologist would be a better resource than a surgeon, and an attorney who specializes in elder law would be better than your corporate lawyer brother-in-law. Forms throughout this book provide the information professionals will need to help you.

Although caregivers are the primary audience for this book, the elderly may find it even more useful, especially those who wish to get their affairs in order. Unless a medical condition has robbed them of competency, the elderly will likely be directly involved in the planning and decision making that affects them. They are as concerned about their own safety and security as any caregiver. As much as this book is about issues that affect them, it is for them as well.

Chapter 1

Caregiving and the Elderly

"Now what do I do?" When you suddenly find yourself in the position of caring or making decisions for an elderly person—whether a parent, relative, or friend—this is usually the first question.

Being a caregiver can be stressful, especially when the obligation arises unexpectedly, such as when a sudden illness or incapacity strikes, or a family situation spins out of control. The issues are complex, the expectations are vague, the legal and medical terms are new, and the information needed to make decisions can be difficult to find.

The best way to begin is to collect and organize the elderly person's essential information, namely, documentation on his or her finances, housing, and healthcare. These documents can help you establish a firm base for decision making. From there you can begin to plan for the future, explore community resources, and select any professional advisors you may need.

Eldercare

Today, the baby-boom, or "sandwich," generation is simultaneously caring for the old and the young. In fact, CNN estimates that by 2002, adults in the United States will be caring for more elderly people than children. However, caring for the elderly is fundamentally different from caring for children. The complexity of the issues and the number of choices involved make caring for the elderly far more demanding—physically, emotionally, and financially.

Children are born completely dependent on their parents. They evolve toward independence over several decades. The elderly move in the opposite direction—from independence to dependence—over several decades. Both the young and the old may require the same basic physical care, such as bathing, dressing, and feeding, but in the case of the elderly, there are additional responsibilities, such as handling financial and housing decisions that were once made independently.

The parent-child relationship is well understood. Our society stresses the welfare of the family and supports parental control over the child's economic, emotional, and educational development. With childcare, we know who is in charge (the parents) and what the objective is (to raise mature adults).

When it comes to eldercare, it is not always clear who is in charge. The elderly person, his or her spouse, an adult child, a social worker, an insurer, the medical community, the courts—the number of people involved can make the situation seem daunting, even frustrating. In addition, the objective may not be clear or, for that matter, shared by all parties. In a medical crisis, for example, objectives may include the elderly person's comfort, dignity, financial standing, or quality of life. Housing objectives could include living alone, living alone with home care, moving in with a sibling, getting into a nursing home, or staying out of a nursing home.

Because uncertainty surrounds the issues of who is in charge and what the objectives are, the decision-making process is not always rational, and good advice is often hard to come by. Furthermore, each situation may be aggravated by any number of factors, such as geographic distance, financial resources, and healthcare rules that affect payment or treatment options. Plus, there is always the need to consider the elderly person's physical and mental condition, living situation, religious views, and the needs of his or her spouse.

Three Elements of Caregiving

There are three factors caregivers must consider in every situation:
1. The elderly person's immediate needs
2. Any and all services available to meet those needs
3. Financial resources available to pay for those services

Identifying Needs
In this book, the word "needs" refers to the physical, mental, emotional, financial, and social condition of the elderly. It involves where they will live, how they will be cared for, and how their medical care will be provided. This book will help you identify and address an elderly person's needs.

Meeting Needs
Once you identify a need, you must find a way to address it. The caregiver and family may be able to provide some services (such as help with bathing, dressing, and grocery shopping), while the community might provide others (such as medical, legal, housing, and general assistance services). Often, the best or most appropriate means are not available, and alternatives must be found. This

book will tell you how to find and evaluate services, and locate alternatives when necessary.

Paying for Services
Meeting the needs of the elderly costs money. Even services performed by family members, such as grocery shopping, can cost time and money. While Medicare covers most acute care medical expenses, and Medicaid may cover certain long-term care expenses, third-party payments are generally the exception, not the rule. This means that even if a service is available, the elderly person and his or her family may not be able to afford it. This book will help you and your family identify your financial resources as well as other care options when these resources are not sufficient.

The following chapters will help you get organized and collect the information you need to make sound, informed decisions. They explain why certain information is important and how you can use that information to best care for an elderly person. The word "care" is used in a broad sense. It may mean dressing, feeding, and so forth, or even something as simple as explaining a tax form or helping with a list of medications.

Chapter 2

Making a Financial Assessment

As a caregiver, it's your job to understand the elderly person's financial situation. Whether a medical crisis has occurred or the elderly person is simply having trouble making ends meet, you must determine if he or she can maintain financial independence. A detailed financial assessment is usually the basis for all other caregiving decisions.

The Four-Step Process

A financial assessment includes four steps:

1. Develop a comprehensive picture of the elderly person's financial position.

2. Determine if the person understands his or her financial position and can manage his or her financial affairs.

3. Determine if the elderly person can live independently without financial or finance-management assistance.

4. Decide who will manage the elderly person's financial affairs if he or she cannot.

Step 1

To complete this step, use the *Vital Information Form* beginning on page 9 and the *Financial Worksheets* on pages 39–54.

The first step of the financial assessment is the most difficult, but it is critical. All financial decisions will be based on this information. Therefore, it must be completed as thoroughly and accurately as possible—and updated regularly. This is not a quick and easy process. Even with the full cooperation of the elderly person, which you are unlikely to have, it will take time. Making phone calls, writing letters, dealing with banks and government agencies, and going through documents, statements, bills, and legal forms—there is a lot to do. You may need the help of lawyers, social workers, real estate agents, or insurance agents to complete this step.

Lack of Cooperation

Don't expect full cooperation from the elderly. A financial assessment is an invasive, and often threatening, process. Even the most mentally competent elderly may resist. They may not see the need for it, or they may view it as an attempt to rob them of their money or independence. Family members may also be uncooperative or suspicious of your motives. Some won't have the time to cooperate; others may worry that you'll uncover something that involves them.

Often, an elderly man's lack of cooperation is rooted in his role as provider and financial decision maker. It can be difficult for older men to entrust financial matters to others, especially their wives or daughters, who are the most likely caregivers. For elderly women, especially those

3

recently widowed, lack of knowledge or lack of trust usually results in a lack of cooperation. Whether because of pride, stubbornness, or a failure to grasp the reality of their situation, obtaining financial information from the elderly takes time and persistence.

Problems with Money Management

During the financial assessment, you may uncover evidence of fraud or careless spending that raises a host of unexpected issues. Be alert for warning signals, such as large checks made out to "cash," insurance companies, financial planners, and lottery or sweepstakes companies, as well as the purchase of unnecessary and inappropriate products, especially through home shopping channels.

The fact-gathering process will tell you if the elderly have recently changed their spending habits and, in some cases, who their "financial advisors and beneficiaries" are. Because of emotional insecurity, questionable financial judgment, or diminished capacity, the elderly may be at high risk for fraud. Often, the size of a check, rather than the recipient's name, should raise concern. An unusually large check for a home-remodeling project, for example, may well be appropriate and explainable, but the elderly person's explanation will tell you a lot about his or her ability to manage money.

Steps 2 and 3

Once you've completed the *Vital Information Form* and *Financial Worksheets,* you must determine if the elderly person understands his or her financial situation, can manage his or her own affairs, and has the resources to live independently. Steps 2 and 3 can be pursued simultaneously, but the issues each deals with are quite different and should not be confused. Step 2 assesses whether the elderly person understands his or her financial situation and has the mental capacity to

manage it prudently. Step 3 determines whether the person's financial resources are sufficient.

It's important to keep these issues separate. Let's say that a new widow doesn't understand her financial position because her husband handled all financial matters. At first it appears that she needs someone to handle her finances. However, once they are explained to her, it turns out she is able to manage her affairs quite well. This is Step 2. In Step 3, however, it becomes apparent that she doesn't have enough money to continue living alone in her home. By dealing with these issues separately, you can see that while she doesn't need help managing her finances, she does need financial support.

Planning for the Future

Although a financial assessment focuses on today's financial resources, you should consider the person's future financial situation as well. For example, most financial assistance and entitlement programs have minimum or set criteria for eligibility. Therefore, a caregiver must consider assets and liabilities (listed on the *Financial Worksheets*) if the elderly person is to qualify for Medicaid, subsidized housing, or other financial assistance in the future. In these areas, it is best to seek the advice of a competent elderlaw attorney or financial advisor. Mistakes can turn into ineligibility for certain types of financial assistance.

Lifestyle Changes

Because the goal is to maintain the elderly person's financial well-being now and in the future, lifestyle changes may be necessary. Keep a record of as many expenditures as possible. Take advantage of discounts for meals, shopping, travel, and entertainment. Plan ahead to minimize unreimbursed medical costs. Take advantage of free services available to the elderly through your Area Agency on Aging or its local equivalent.

Step 4

If the elderly person needs help managing finances, the level of assistance should be appropriate for his or her needs. Some elderly people need only partial assistance. For example, many are able to manage day-to-day financial transactions but are befuddled by investment decisions. Others may be comfortable managing all of their finances but may need someone else to write checks and keep records because arthritic hands prevent them from doing so.

If an elderly person needs only partial assistance—someone to sign checks, make sure taxes are paid, and so forth—the whole family should decide who will provide that assistance. The elderly person's consent is essential, and there should be no question about his or her ability to understand what is happening. Above all, trust is key. There should be no mingling of an elderly person's funds or assets with those of the caregiver or financial advisor.

Durable Power of Attorney

During the financial assessment, you might suggest getting a durable power of attorney as a way to provide partial assistance and plan for the future. A durable power of attorney (discussed in chapter 6) is a legally binding document executed by an elderly person when he or she is mentally competent. It grants another person the authority to make decisions on the elderly person's behalf and can be drafted to take effect only when the elderly person becomes incompetent. It might also limit the nature of decisions that can be made.

A durable power of attorney is an excellent way to transfer partial or total decision-making power.

It is quick, easy, inexpensive, and private. The alternative is a legal guardianship proceeding, which is slow, difficult, expensive, and public. From the standpoint of the elderly, a durable power of attorney may be preferable to a guardianship proceeding because it allows the elderly, rather than a judge, to decide who will make decisions on their behalf when they are no longer able.

If a power of attorney does not exist, and the elderly person suddenly becomes incompetent (as the result of a stroke, for example), you should consult an elderlaw attorney about a guardianship proceeding. It's important not to disrupt the elderly person's care; therefore, decisions must be made on his or her behalf.

Questions of Competence

If the financial assessment raises questions about the person's legal competence, seek professional assistance. In many situations, the elderly person's incompetence may appear self-evident. Be aware, however, that "competency" is a legal concept governed by state law.

If there's no durable power of attorney in place, and if the elderly person becomes unable to manage his or her financial affairs, it's generally best to have a legal guardian appointed. In most cases, this requires time and a knowledgeable attorney. Nevertheless, it's better than an informal arrangement among family members, especially if the elderly person isn't aware that his or her affairs have been effectively taken over by others, or if there's a chance that someone in the family will object to a self-appointed guardian.

Collecting Vital Information

What You Need to Know

Before you begin your financial assessment, you need to verify important sources of information about the elderly person. To do this, you can use the *Vital Information Form* beginning on page 9. Because this form is critical to financial decision making, it should be completed and updated periodically for every elderly person, regardless of his or her current situation.

In addition to helping you gather key information, the *Vital Information Form* will tell you where to go if you need help clarifying that information. Too often, a caregiver will be satisfied to locate a long-term care insurance policy but will not take the time to fully understand the types of coverage, application deadlines, and any preconditions that must be satisfied.

Remember, no one understands it all, and you won't either. Seek help. If you can't afford to hire a professional, see if a qualified neighbor, church member, or friend can answer your questions. Gathering the information will take time—it may even seem like a waste of time if there are other pressing problems—but you will be better equipped to understand and assist in handling the elderly person's financial affairs.

If you are an elderly person, you shouldn't wait for someone else to begin this process. If you don't want to share this information with others, complete the form anyway and keep it in a safe place. That way, if you need someone else to take over your affairs in the future, the information will help make a smoother transition. It will also help professionals, such as your attorney, financial advisor, or insurance consultant, to assist you in managing your affairs. Even if the *Vital Information Form* is not disclosed until after your death, it will make things easier for your surviving spouse and family. For example, it may help lower estate administration fees by providing much of the information your family would need to close your estate.

How to Use the *Vital Information Form*

The checklist on page 7 is a list of the information that will appear on the *Vital Information Form*. It tells you which documents you will need to collect. The actual worksheet (beginning on page 9) will give you space to record this information. It will also provide detailed instructions and explanations. Note: The *Vital Information Form* is fairly comprehensive, so many items won't apply to your situation. You may end up with a number of blank lines after you're finished.

Some information will come to you by word of mouth, and if this is all you have, use it. But remember, verbal reports are often unreliable. Eventually you will need the official information, so it's important to get copies of documents despite the extra time and money involved. When in doubt about whether to get a document, get it. For official documents, such as birth and death certificates, get multiple copies with the raised official governmental seal. It will cost more, but some documents aren't official without the seal. (See also Collecting Key Documents on page 192.)

Vital Information Checklist

The following is a list of categories included in the *Vital Information Form* beginning on page 9. This list is not a substitute for the form; it is simply a quick reference to the information you'll need to assess an elderly person's financial situation.

Name
____ Current name
____ Maiden name
____ Other names
    ____ Nicknames
    ____ Previous married names
____ Computer names

Identification
____ Social Security card
____ Passport
____ Driver's license
____ Medicare claim number
____ Birth certificate
____ Marriage certificate
____ VA claim number or honorable
      discharge certificate
____ Spouse's death certificate
____ Spouse's Social Security number
____ Naturalization papers
____ Adoption papers
____ Divorce papers or decree
____ Employer identification number

Financial Information
____ Checking accounts
    ____ Banks
    ____ Credit unions
    ____ Brokerage
    ____ Lines of credit
____ Savings accounts
    ____ Banks
    ____ Credit unions
____ CDs (certificates of deposit) or savings certificates
____ Savings bonds
____ Money market accounts

____ Publicly traded bonds and notes
____ Publicly traded stock certificates
____ Mutual fund shares
____ IRAs (individual retirement accounts)
____ Keogh-type plans
____ 401(k) or 403(b) plans
____ Insurance policies (with equity or cash value)
____ Rights to receive money
    ____ Social Security
    ____ Pension plans
    ____ Annuity contracts
    ____ Trust funds
    ____ Loans/notes receivable
    ____ Government programs
    ____ Miscellaneous
____ Real estate owned
    ____ Primary residence
    ____ Secondary residence
    ____ Other residences
    ____ Rental property
    ____ Time share
    ____ Undeveloped land
    ____ Cemetery plot
____ Personal property
    ____ Automobiles
    ____ Other items requiring ownership documents
    ____ Special collections
    ____ Personal possessions
____ Insurance
    ____ Whole life
    ____ Term life
    ____ Group life
    ____ Automobile
    ____ Homeowners
    ____ Renters

_____ Umbrella
_____ Health insurance supplement/
Medigap/major medical
_____ Dental
_____ Long-term care
_____ Professional liability tail coverage
_____ Business
_____ Money owed
_____ Mortgages
_____ Home equity loans
_____ Automobile loans/leases

_____ Other secured loans
_____ Margin loans
_____ Loans against cash value of insurance
_____ Business loans
_____ Unsecured loans
_____ Credit card debt
_____ Miscellaneous expenses
_____ Assets owned by only one spouse
_____ Asset transferred within the last five years

VITAL INFORMATION FORM

It's important to fill out these first few lines in case you are unable or unavailable to pass the information on to others. The date is important for knowing when the information was last updated, since it will change over time, and the location of the supporting documents is vital. While the inventory is most accurate when completed by the elderly person, it's usually prepared by a caregiver. (The elderly often won't see the need for it because they know—or think they know—all the relevant facts.)

Vital Information for (name) _____

Completed by _____

Date completed _____

Location of documents _____

_____

NAME

This section helps identify the name the elderly person was given at birth, as well as other names he or she may have used in his or her lifetime. Some people use their first name, some their second, and some just an initial. Preferences like this can change over time.

The name on the birth certificate may be different from the name on the Social Security card. As you look through legal and financial documents, it may help to know that Suzanne Smith, Elizabeth Suzanne Smith, Mrs. Thomas Smith, Suzanne Jones, Elizabeth S. Jones, Suzanne Jones-Smith, and Mrs. Suzanne Wilson are all the same person. You might also note if "Suzanne" has been spelled "Susanne" or "Suzonne" at different points in her life. Spelling variations are common among the elderly, especially among those who have immigrated to the United States. Also, women are likely to use several last names, which may include their maiden name, various married names, or hyphenated names.

With the proliferation of computer services, on-line trading, and e-mail, many people have taken online names that are completely different from their given names. Information on accounts belonging to the elderly may be scattered all over the Internet and might only be accessed online. Although passwords and personal identification numbers (PINs) should only be given out in unusual situations, the completion of this form may be one of those situations. To track down this information later would be very difficult, and vital information could be lost forever.

Name on birth certificate _____

Name on Social Security card, or with the Social Security Administration

_____

Maiden name _____

Other names (previous marriages, stage names, other spellings, nicknames)

_____

Computer names, passwords, and PINs

_____

IDENTIFICATION

This section continues to focus on the elderly person's identity. Again, some of this information—such as a Social Security number—is only given out in unusual situations, but filling out this form may be one of those situations.

A passport or driver's license (even one that has expired) will provide photo identification, which could be useful in the most unexpected circumstances. For example, an elderly person may not be allowed on a domestic airline without a photo ID. (See also Collecting Key Documents on page 192.)

The spouse's death certificate is included here because survivors may not be entitled to benefits unless they can prove the identity and death of their spouse. Other information will be important if official documentation is required in the future.

Some elderly people will have an employer identification number, especially with the increasing number of self-employed individuals and home offices. If there is a possibility that the elderly person may have had employees, get the employer identification number.

Social Security number_____
Get a copy of the card.

Passport number_____
Get a copy of the passport.

Driver's license number _____
Get a copy of the current or last license.

Medicare claim number _____
Get a copy of the card.

Birth certificate_____
If not receiving Social Security, get several copies of the certificate.

Marriage certificate _____

VA claim number _____

Honorable discharge certificate _____

Death certificate of spouse _____

Social Security number of spouse_____

Naturalization papers_____

Adoption papers_____

Divorce papers, settlement agreements, court orders _____

_____

Employer identification number_____

FINANCIAL INFORMATION

This section focuses mainly on the elderly person's financial assets, starting with checking and savings accounts.

Note that each entry is numbered, so if there isn't enough room on the form or if you wish to record additional information, continue on a separate sheet of paper. Simply reference the correct number. Also, this form generally doesn't ask for dollar amounts, such as how much money is in a checking account or mutual fund. This information will be entered later on the *Financial Worksheets.*

Knowing the location of accessible cash is as important as knowing who has access to it, where the records are, and whether any funds (like Social Security checks or loan payments) are automatically deposited or withdrawn from the account. It's critical to know if anyone else has access to an account, whether by title (as in a joint checking account) or as an authorized signer (through a power of attorney, for example). If so, someone else may claim the assets. It's also important to know if anyone has access to debit or ATM cards that could reduce the amount of money in the account. Other than ATM cards, which are controlled by a PIN or password, access to bank accounts usually can only occur by changing the user's signature cards.

Don't forget to check for Christmas Club accounts or cash stashed away in a drawer, safe, or safety deposit box. Many elderly people like to have cash around, and they tend to rely on the simple "investment" methods they grew up with. You may find substantial amounts of cash hidden away or sitting in a low- or non-interest-bearing account.

Two important accounts are not listed on this worksheet—foreign bank accounts and business accounts. If these exist, write the relevant information on a separate sheet of paper and attach it to the worksheet. For foreign accounts, an account number and password are normally needed to access funds. For a small business account, the elderly person may still be listed on the account, even if he or she retired or is no longer actively involved in the business. Because liability or estate problems could come up later on, the person's name should be removed from the account if he or she is no longer an active participant.

1. Checking accounts

a. Bank _____ Branch _____ Account number _____

Other authorized signers _____

Who has checkbook? _____ Who has statements? _____

Direct deposits? _____ Direct withdrawals? _____

Overdraft protection? _____ ATM or debit card? _____

b. Bank _____ Branch _____ Account number _____

Other authorized signers _____

Who has checkbook? _____ Who has statements? _____

Direct deposits? _____ Direct withdrawals? _____

Overdraft protection? _____ ATM or debit card? _____

c. Credit union _____ Member number _____

Other authorized signers _____

Who has checkbook? _____ Who has statements? _____

Direct deposits? _____ Direct withdrawals? _____

Overdraft protection? _____ ATM or debit card? _____

d. Brokerage _____ Account number _____

Broker name _____ Margin account? _____

Other authorized signers _____

Who has checkbook? _____ Who has statements? _____

Direct deposits? _____ Direct withdrawals? _____

e. Line of credit: Issuer _____ Account number _____

Other authorized signers _____

Who has checkbook? _____ Who has statements? _____

Direct deposits? _____ Direct withdrawals? _____

2. Savings accounts

a. Bank _____ Branch _____ Account number _____

Other authorized signers _____

Who has passbook? _____ Who has statements? _____

Direct deposits? _____ Direct withdrawals? _____

b. Credit union _____ Member number _____

Other authorized signers _____

Who has passbook? _____ Who has statements? _____

Direct deposits? _____ Direct withdrawals? _____

3. CDs (certificates of deposit) or savings certificates

When completing numbers 3 and 4, keep in mind that the elderly are likely to keep their CDs or savings bonds in a desk, a safe, or a safety deposit box. It is unlikely that these documents will be held by a brokerage firm or third party.

a. Bank _____ Branch _____ Certificate number _____

Amount _____ Interest rate _____ Maturity date _____

Who has CD? _____ Renewal date _____

Names (if held in joint name) _____

b. Bank _____ Branch _____ Certificate number _____

Amount _____ Interest rate _____ Maturity date _____

Who has CD? _____ Renewal date _____

Names (if held in joint name) _____

c. Bank _____ Branch_____ Certificate number _____

Amount _____ Interest rate _____ Maturity date _____

Who has CD? _____ Renewal date_____

Names (if held in joint name) _____

d. Bank_____ Branch_____ Certificate number _____

Amount _____ Interest rate _____ Maturity date _____

Who has CD? _____ Renewal date_____

Names (if held in joint name) _____

4. Savings bonds

a. Number on bond_____ Face amount _____

Maturity date_____ Who had bond? _____

Names (if held in joint name) _____

b. Number on bond _____ Face amount _____

Maturity date_____ Who had bond? _____

Names (if held in joint name) _____

Numbers 5 through 13 focus on assets that generate cash, can be easily converted to cash, or represent the right to receive funds. Elderly people may have the right to receive funds for several reasons:

- Federal law (Social Security)
- Their work history or their spouse's work history (pension)
- They have invested money in the past to receive a guaranteed payment in the future (such as an annuity contract)

- Family arrangement (such as each child paying $100 a month for a parent's support)

With some assets, it's important to find out (1) if the benefits have been applied for and (2) if all the conditions for receiving these benefits have been met. Next, you must determine what conditions are necessary for continued payment, noting anything that could change (and especially increase) the benefit level. For example, trust payments may change if marital status changes or when a person reaches a certain age. As with any right to receive money, you must understand the terms for payment. If you do not, you should seek the help of an attorney or accountant.

When you look at assets that generate cash, remember that stocks and bonds may be held by the elderly person or his or her broker. If stocks are held by the elderly person, find out if the company has a dividend reinvestment program. This could mean that additional assets exist. It could also mean that money is automatically withdrawn from the elderly person's account to acquire more stock.

Number 13 lists several examples of money that the elderly person may have received within the last thirty-six months. These are often overlooked because they are not treated as income for tax purposes. However, many federal and state programs will consider these funds when deciding if an elderly person is eligible for certain benefits.

Employment contracts, stock option plans, deferred compensation arrangements, profit-sharing agreements, partnerships (general or limited), and accounts receivable (payments due) are not included on this worksheet. If applicable, they should be included on a separate sheet of paper. (You may need to consult a professional to fully understand the elderly person's rights and obligations.)

5. Money market accounts

a. Institution or company _____

Account number_____

Contact person_____ Direct deposits?_____

Other authorized signers _____

b. Institution or company _____

Account number_____

Contact person_____ Direct deposits?_____

Other authorized signers _____

A Family Caregiver's Guide to Planning and Decision Making for the Elderly © 1999 James A. Wilkinson

6. Publicly traded bonds and notes

a. Issuer _____ Face value _____

CUSIP number _____ Maturity date _____

Interest payment dates_____ Coupon bond? _____

Fixed or variable rate? _____ Who holds bond?_____

Names (if held in joint name)_____

b. Issuer_____ Face value _____

CUSIP number _____ Maturity date _____

Interest payment dates_____ Coupon bond? _____

Fixed or variable rate? _____ Who holds bond?_____

Names (if held in joint name)_____

c. Issuer _____ Face value _____

CUSIP number _____ Maturity date _____

Interest payment dates_____ Coupon bond? _____

Fixed or variable rate? _____ Who holds bond?_____

Names (if held in joint name)_____

7. Publicly traded stock certificates

a. Company _____

Number of shares _____

Who holds shares? _____

Names (if held in joint name)_____

Date purchased _____ Price at acquisition_____

A Family Caregiver's Guide to Planning and Decision Making for the Elderly © 1999 James A. Wilkinson

b. Company_____

Number of shares _____

Who holds shares? _____

Names (if held in joint name)_____

Date purchased _____ Price at acquisition_____

c. Company_____

Number of shares _____

Who holds shares? _____

Names (if held in joint name)_____

Date purchased _____ Price at acquisition_____

d. Company_____

Number of shares _____

Who holds shares? _____

Names (if held in joint name)_____

Date purchased _____ Price at acquisition_____

e. Company_____

Number of shares _____

Who holds shares? _____

Names (if held in joint name)_____

Date purchased _____ Price at acquisition_____

8. Mutual fund shares

a. Fund name _____

Number of shares _____ Account number _____

Joint name or restrictions?_____

Date purchased _____ Price at acquisition_____

b. Fund name _____

Number of shares _____ Account number _____

Joint name or restrictions?_____

Date purchased _____ Price at acquisition_____

c. Fund name _____

Number of shares _____ Account number _____

Joint name or restrictions?_____

Date purchased _____ Price at acquisition_____

9. IRAs (individual retirement accounts)

a. Institution _____ Account number_____

Contact person _____

Investments (stocks, fixed-income) _____

b. Institution _____ Account number_____

Contact person _____

Investments (stocks, fixed-income) _____

c. Institution _____ Account number_____

Contact person _____

Investments (stocks, fixed-income) _____

d. Institution_____ Account number_____

Contact person _____

Investments (stocks, fixed-income) _____

10. Keogh-type plans

a. Institution_____ Account number_____

Contact person _____

Investments (stocks, fixed-income) _____

b. Institution_____ Account number_____

Contact person _____

Investments (stocks, fixed-income) _____

c. Institution_____ Account number_____

Contact person _____

Investments (stocks, fixed-income) _____

11. 401(k) or 403(b) plans

a. Institution_____ Account number_____

Contact person _____

Company match _____

Investments (stocks, fixed-income) _____

b. Institution_____ Account number_____

Contact person _____

Company match _____

Investments (stocks, fixed-income) _____

c. Institution _____ Account number_____

Contact person _____

Company match _____

Investments (stocks, fixed-income) _____

12. Insurance policies (with equity or cash value)

a. Institution _____

Policy number and type_____

Death benefit_____ Paid-up additions_____ Cash surrender value _____

b. Institution _____

Policy number and type_____

Death benefit_____ Paid-up additions_____ Cash surrender value _____

c. Institution _____

Policy number and type_____

Death benefit_____ Paid-up additions_____ Cash surrender value _____

13. Rights to receive money (or money received within the last twelve months)

a. Social Security

Eligible for? yes • no   Applied for? yes • no   Receiving? yes • no

Direct deposit? yes • no   Name of financial institution _____

b. Pension plans

Payer _____ Reference number _____

Type of plan _____ Joint/survivor option? _____

Payer _____ Reference number _____

Type of plan _____ Joint/survivor option? _____

c. Annuity contracts

Payer _____ Contact person or agent _____

Reference number _____ Payment dates _____

Payer _____ Contact person or agent _____

Reference number _____ Payment dates _____

d. Trust funds

Payer _____ Contact person or trustee _____

Reference number _____ Payment dates _____

e. Loans/notes receivable

Obligor _____ Interest rate _____

Security _____ Payment dates _____

Location of contract or note _____ Due date _____

Obligor _____ Interest rate _____

Security _____ Payment dates _____

Location of contract or note _____ Due date _____

f. Government programs (such as workers' compensation)

Program _____ Contact person _____

Type _____ Payment dates _____

Program _____ Contact person _____

Type _____ Payment dates _____

g. Inheritance (over $1,000)

From _____ Payment date _____

Amount _____

From _____ Payment date _____

Amount _____

h. Lottery or contest winnings (over $1,000)

Amount _____ Payment date _____

i. Gift money (over $1,000)

Gift from _____ Payment date _____

Amount _____

j. Life insurance proceeds (over $1,000)

Name of the deceased _____

Payment date _____ Amount _____

k. Miscellaneous

Payer _____

Location of contract or note _____

_____

Payer _____

Location of contract or note _____

_____

14. Real estate owned

With real estate, you must determine what is owned, who lives there, where the deeds are, and, if applicable, who the manager or leasing agent is. You will need this information to identify related liabilities (taxes, mortgages, upkeep, management fees) and restrictions on transfer when you complete the *Financial Worksheets*.

a. Primary residence

Address _____ City, state_____

Name(s) on deed _____

Deed location _____ Condo or cooperative?_____

Who is living there? _____

Manager name, if condo or coop_____ Telephone number_____

b. Secondary residence

Address _____ City, state_____

Name(s) on deed _____

Deed location _____ Condo or cooperative?_____

Who is living there? _____

Manager name, if condo or coop_____ Telephone number_____

c. Other residences

Address _____ City, state_____

Name(s) on deed _____

Deed location _____ Condo or cooperative?_____

Who is living there? _____

Manager name, if condo or coop_____ Telephone number_____

d. Rental property

Address _____ City, state_____

Name(s) on deed _____

Deed location _____ Condo or cooperative?_____

Who is living there? _____

Manager name, if condo or coop_____ Telephone number _____

e. Time share

Address _____ City, state_____

Name(s) on time share _____ Use periods _____

Duration _____ Management agent _____

f. Undeveloped land

Address _____ City, state_____

Name(s) on deed _____

Current use _____

g. Cemetery plot

Address _____ City, state_____

Plot location _____

15. Personal property

With personal property, the inventory process has three steps. First, identify items for which there is a "used" market, such as cars, boats, and trailers. (Locate all titles and other ownership papers.) Second, identify any hobbies or collections that may have value to other collectors or dealers. (List each item in each collection, noting its condition, location, and owner.) Third, list personal possessions, room by room.

Although personal property can be videotaped, it is best to have a written list as well. You can simplify the process by listing only unique or special items over an estimated dollar value. Other items, such as cooking supplies, can be listed generically.

The main goal is to identify and inventory any property that could (1) generate income if needed or (2) incur an ongoing expense or obligation if held. Most household items will do neither. However, by recording every item, its location, and its owner, you may avoid ownership disputes among family members later on.

a. Automobiles

Year_____ Make _____ Model_____

Own or lease? _____ Name on title _____

Vehicle identification number _____

Lien holder or loss payee_____

Year_____ Make _____ Model_____

Own or lease? _____ Name on title _____

Vehicle identification number _____

Lien holder or loss payee_____

b. Other items requiring ownership documents (boat, airplane, trailer, and so forth)

_____

_____

_____

c. Special collections (stamps, dolls, guns, coins, jewelry, and so forth)

Item _____ Owner_____ Location_____

Condition _____

Item _____ Owner_____ Location_____

Condition _____

Item _____ Owner_____ Location_____

Condition _____

Item _____ Owner _____ Location _____

Condition _____

d. Personal possessions (by location)

Be as specific as possible. Be sure to include items in storage, being repaired, or borrowed by others. Also note items that have been loaned to the elderly person that will ultimately have to be returned.

_____

_____

_____

_____

_____

_____

_____

_____

_____

_____

_____

_____

_____

_____

16. Insurance

It is important to know what each insurance policy covers, the level of coverage provided, and the preconditions or requirements for making a claim. If you don't fully understand all these areas, you should hire an insurance consultant or financial advisor to assist you.

The elderly are often overinsured in some areas, underinsured in others, and ineligible for some of the benefits they think they have. They tend to pay too much for their insurance and fail to take advantage of discounts that could save them a substantial amount of money.

Be sure to collect all non-healthcare policies and review them for obvious problems, such as the following:

- Deductibles that are too low
- Social Security discounts that have gone unclaimed

- No riders purchased to cover valuables
- No current inventory to support a claim for theft

For life insurance policies, pay particular attention to who owns the policy and who is the beneficiary, especially if this information has recently changed.

Given the limitations on Medicare, the elderly person should have some kind of supplemental major medical or Medigap coverage (unless he or she qualifies for Medicaid).

If you are not sure what Medigap coverage is or what is covered, consult a health insurer. Make sure that both you and the elderly person understand Medicaid "spend down" and asset transfer policies, the services covered by Medicare HMOs, and preexisting condition limitations. With long-term care insurance, note any preconditions for coverage (such as a prior hospital stay, a long waiting period, exclusions for dementia, or payment only if the person is institutionalized).

a. Whole life

Amount _____ Beneficiary _____

Premium due date _____ Company _____

Agent _____ Policy number _____

b. Term life

Amount _____ Beneficiary _____

Premium due date _____ Company _____

Agent _____ Policy number _____

c. Group life

Amount _____ Beneficiary _____

Premium due date _____ Company _____

Agent _____ Policy number _____

d. Automobile

Company _____ Policy number _____

Agent _____ Policy expires _____ Deductibles _____

A Family Caregiver's Guide to Planning and Decision Making for the Elderly © 1999 James A. Wilkinson

e. Homeowners

Company _____ Policy number _____

Agent _____ Policy expires _____ Deductibles _____

f. Renters

Company _____ Policy number _____

Agent _____ Policy expires _____ Deductibles _____

g. Umbrella

Company _____ Policy number _____

Agent _____ Policy expires _____ Deductibles _____

h. Health insurance supplement/Medigap/major medical

Company _____ Policy number _____

Agent _____ Policy expires _____

Deductibles or copayments _____

i. Dental

Company _____ Policy number _____

Agent _____ Policy expires _____

Deductibles or copayments _____

j. Long-term care

Company _____ Policy number _____

Agent _____ Policy expires _____

Deductibles or copayments _____

k. Professional liability tail coverage

Company _____ Policy number _____

Agent _____ Policy expires _____ Deductibles _____

l. Business

Company _____ Policy number _____

Agent _____ Policy expires _____ Deductibles _____

17. Money owed

If the elderly person has taken on loans and other financial obligations, contact his or her creditors to determine the payoff amounts, especially if these loans are secured by property or other collateral. Even if a loan won't be paid off soon, this is an easy way to learn the account's payment status. The amount due can be recorded in the *Financial Worksheets* (page 52).

If the elderly person owes money on certain property, you'll need to know how much money is owed in case you decide to sell it. For example, if $6,000 is owed on a car, and you sell it for only $5,000, all of this money will go to the lender. Furthermore, an additional $1,000 will have to be found to pay off the debt. However, selling the car will save a monthly payment of $350, so it still may be a good idea to sell. The payoff amount needs to be factored into the decision, as well as any prepayment penalties that might apply.

a. Mortgages

Owed to _____ Original amount _____ Interest rate _____

Loan/account number _____ Security _____ Due date _____

b. Home equity loans

Owed to _____ Original amount _____ Interest rate _____

Loan/account number _____ Security _____ Due date _____

c. Automobile loans/leases

Owed to_____ Original amount _____ Interest rate_____

Loan/account number_____ Security _____ Due date _____

d. Other secured loans

Owed to_____ Original amount _____ Interest rate_____

Loan/account number_____ Security _____ Due date _____

e. Margin loans

Owed to_____ Original amount _____ Interest rate_____

Loan/account number_____ Security _____ Due date _____

f. Loans against cash value of insurance

Owed to_____ Original amount _____ Interest rate_____

Loan/account number _____

g. Business loans

Owed to_____ Original amount _____ Interest rate_____

Loan/account number_____ Security _____ Due date _____

h. Unsecured loans

Owed to_____ Original amount _____ Interest rate_____

Loan/account number_____ Security _____ Due date _____

18. Credit card debt

It can be difficult to find out which credit cards have been issued in the elderly person's name. The best way to identify every credit card and balance is to get a banker to run the person's credit history. Many cards carry annual fees and high interest rates, so it's important to close unnecessary cards.

Also, if the person's credit history shows past due amounts or unexplained charges, you should investigate these to be sure that there's no fraud involved or that other family members aren't using the elderly person's credit card.

Issuer _____ Account number _____ Balance _____

Issuer _____ Account number _____ Balance _____

Issuer _____ Account number _____ Balance _____

Issuer _____ Account number _____ Balance _____

Issuer _____ Account number _____ Balance _____

Issuer _____ Account number _____ Balance _____

Issuer _____ Account number _____ Balance _____

Issuer _____ Account number _____ Balance _____

Issuer _____ Account number _____ Balance _____

Issuer _____ Account number _____ Balance _____

19. Miscellaneous expenses

The *Financial Worksheets* will help you identify routine expenses for housing, taxes, food, medical care, clothing, transportation, personal possessions, and donations or contributions. Thus, there is no need to enter them here. Instead, you will enter only miscellaneous expenses, such as unfulfilled pledges, items that have been ordered but not fully paid for, and contests or lotteries.

Type _____ Due date(s) _____ Amount _____

Type _____ Due date(s) _____ Amount _____

Type _____ Due date(s) _____ Amount _____

Type _____ Due date(s) _____ Amount _____

Type _____ Due date(s) _____ Amount _____

20. Assets owned by only one spouse

If the elderly person has a living spouse, identify assets that are owned exclusively by one partner or the other. (It is assumed that all other assets listed on this worksheet are owned jointly unless otherwise shown.)

The ownership of assets becomes an issue when determining eligibility for Medicaid. Medicaid is complex, and the rules vary from state to state. You will need the help of an experienced elderlaw attorney when planning for Medicaid. This section is designed to help you collect some of the information the attorney will need to advise you.

In a marriage, most things are acquired and owned jointly. When one partner dies, ownership automatically passes to the survivor. Note that ownership is different than use. For example, jewelry may be purchased and worn only by the wife, and golf clubs may be purchased and used only by the husband, but these items would still be owned jointly.

Typically, only financial instruments, such as stock, or big-ticket items that require title or ownership papers, such as cars, are owned individually.

Wife's individually owned assets

_____

_____

_____

_____

_____

_____

_____

Husband's individually owned assets

_____

_____

_____

_____

_____

_____

_____

21. Assets transferred within the last five years

This section also relates to Medicaid eligibility. When an elderly person applies for Medicaid, reviewers look to see if certain assets were transferred (sold or given away) during some period prior to the date of application. While in many states the period is three years, it can be as many as five years. If you do not know what your state's "look back" period is, contact an elderlaw attorney.

Use this section to collect information that an accountant, elderlaw attorney, or financial planner will need to fill out Medicaid forms and determine if there is an eligibility problem. Since small transfers should not affect eligibility, record only those assets that (1) had a fair market value over $2,000 and (2) were given away or sold for substantially less than the fair market value within the applicable "look back" period. A separate record should be kept of all transfers, regardless of value.

Asset transferred_____ Date transferred _____

To whom transferred _____

Amount or consideration received _____

Asset transferred_____ Date transferred _____

To whom transferred _____

Amount or consideration received _____

Asset transferred_____ Date transferred _____

To whom transferred _____

Amount or consideration received _____

Asset transferred_____ Date transferred _____

To whom transferred _____

Amount or consideration received _____

Asset transferred_____ Date transferred _____

To whom transferred _____

Amount or consideration received _____

Understanding Finances

What You Need to Know

To evaluate an elderly person's financial position, use the *Financial Worksheets* beginning on page 39. These worksheets will help you assess the person's finances, particularly his or her cash flow over a specific time period. This will allow you to:

- Make sure that the elderly person's income is enough to cover his or her expenses.
- Determine which assets can be converted to cash in an emergency.
- Get a sense of whether the elderly person needs help managing his or her financial affairs.

Before You Begin …

Once the *Vital Information Form* (pages 9–33) is complete, it will help if you fill out the *Monthly Expense Forms* (pages 36–37) and *Medical Charges and Payments Form* (page 38) before moving on to the *Financial Worksheets.*

The *Monthly Expense Forms* will help you record information about the elderly person's routine monthly expenses. The first form tracks monthly payments and bills, such as rent and utilities. The second tracks daily cash expenditures, such as gasoline, groceries, medications, and restaurant meals. Knowing how, when, and where the elderly person's money is spent will help you complete the financial assessment—and it will help the elderly avoid the anxiety of not remembering where their cash went.

The *Medical Charges and Payments Form* tracks medical charges and payments. This form should be updated continuously, since new charges are often incurred before previous charges are settled by the insurance company. It breaks payments into separate categories, so overcharges can be easily detected.

Once you have completed these forms, the *Financial Worksheets* are easy to do. Except for certain routine expenses, virtually all the information can be taken directly from the *Vital Information Form* and the *Monthly Expense Forms.*

How to Use the *Financial Worksheets*

There are two *Financial Worksheets.* Part 1 compares income and expenses over a specific time period, usually one month. Part 2 evaluates other assets and liabilities.

Although there are many categories listed on each worksheet, the elderly person is unlikely to have expenses or sources of income in every category. Therefore, you might end up with only a few completed entries on each worksheet.

The *Financial Worksheets* can be used for a single person or for a couple. For a couple, look at their income and expenses separately to prepare for possible events in the future. For example, if a couple is living comfortably in their own home when the husband dies, housing expenses would stay the same, but the widow's Social Security and pension benefits would decrease significantly. She may no longer be able to afford the home and might be forced to sell off some assets or move out.

The *Financial Worksheets* are not traditional balance sheets, which determine a person's net worth as of a given day. While balance sheets can be important, especially for Medicaid and other programs, caregivers are less interested in an elderly person's worth on any given day than with whether he or she has enough money to pay monthly bills.

Also, traditional balance sheets give equal weight to all assets: $50,000 in the bank has the same value as a home worth $50,000. But a home creates ongoing expenses for taxes, maintenance, and utilities. Unless the home is to be mortgaged, rented, or sold in the near future, it's easier for caregivers to think of it as a liability, not an asset.

These worksheets won't tell you what to do about an elderly person's financial situation, but they will help you assess the situation realistically, identifying expenses that are inordinately high or assets that could be converted to cash in an emergency. If you're confused or you think there's a problem after completing the *Financial Worksheets,* seek professional assistance from a financial planner, accountant, or elderlaw attorney.

How to Use the
Monthly Expense Forms

The following forms will help you gather information you will need for the *Financial Worksheets.* Because this information will change from month to month, make copies of each form and use a new one every month.

Two examples are listed on the *Bill Payments* form. Notice that the full amount has been paid on one bill, and a partial amount on the other. If "budget" or partial payments are made, be sure to keep track of the total amount due, because these will ultimately have to be paid.

For bill payments, refer to the original invoices to get accurate amounts. For cash transactions, however, you'll need to get in the habit of asking for (and keeping) store receipts. Bill payments may require only one or two entries a month, whenever checks are written. Cash transactions, on the other hand, should be entered daily, if possible, since it's hard to remember a week or two later exactly where that cash was spent. Use the "comments" column to note what the cash was used for—groceries, restaurants, entertainment, clothing, and so forth.

Monthly Expense Form: BILL PAYMENTS for the month of _____

Provider	Date received	Amount due	Date due	Amount paid	Date paid (cash or check)	Balance due
Bell Atlantic	12/6	$33.45	12/22	$33.45	12/15 Chk #1325	0
Gas Company	12/7	$245.30	12/25	$80.00	12/21 Chk #1326	$165.30
_____	_____	_____	_____	_____	_____	_____
_____	_____	_____	_____	_____	_____	_____
_____	_____	_____	_____	_____	_____	_____
_____	_____	_____	_____	_____	_____	_____
_____	_____	_____	_____	_____	_____	_____
_____	_____	_____	_____	_____	_____	_____
_____	_____	_____	_____	_____	_____	_____
_____	_____	_____	_____	_____	_____	_____
_____	_____	_____	_____	_____	_____	_____
_____	_____	_____	_____	_____	_____	_____
_____	_____	_____	_____	_____	_____	_____
_____	_____	_____	_____	_____	_____	_____
_____	_____	_____	_____	_____	_____	_____
_____	_____	_____	_____	_____	_____	_____
_____	_____	_____	_____	_____	_____	_____
_____	_____	_____	_____	_____	_____	_____
_____	_____	_____	_____	_____	_____	_____

Monthly Expense Form: CASH TRANSACTIONS for the month of _____

Date	Cash paid	Paid to	Comments
_____	_____	_____	_____
_____	_____	_____	_____
_____	_____	_____	_____
_____	_____	_____	_____
_____	_____	_____	_____
_____	_____	_____	_____
_____	_____	_____	_____
_____	_____	_____	_____
_____	_____	_____	_____
_____	_____	_____	_____
_____	_____	_____	_____
_____	_____	_____	_____
_____	_____	_____	_____
_____	_____	_____	_____
_____	_____	_____	_____
_____	_____	_____	_____
_____	_____	_____	_____
_____	_____	_____	_____
_____	_____	_____	_____
_____	_____	_____	_____
_____	_____	_____	_____
_____	_____	_____	_____
_____	_____	_____	_____
_____	_____	_____	_____

A Family Caregiver's Guide to Planning and Decision Making for the Elderly © 1999 James A. Wilkinson

MEDICAL CHARGES AND PAYMENTS FORM

There are two main reasons to track charges and payments for medical care:

1. To keep track of what's been billed, what's been paid, and what you owe for medical treatment.

2. To be able to look at medical charges over several months so you can estimate the average monthly cost of medical care (you will need this information for the *Financial Worksheets*).

Use this form to record any copayments, deductibles, and payments that the elderly person makes, as well as payments by Medicare, Medicaid, or medical insurance. Remember, while many providers will accept an insurance payment as payment in full, claims that are denied may become the elderly person's obligation. Update this form after each new medical charge for easy reconciliation of charges and payments.

Keep copies of all charges, correspondence, and statements. Make an effort to learn the billing codes, and know the person's rights of appeal. Aggressively contest inappropriate charges, denials based upon lack of support, and requests for payment when the charge exceeds "usual and customary charge." Finally, do not hesitate to negotiate payment terms with a healthcare provider.

Provider or product_____ Date_____

Copayment or amount paid toward deductible _____

Amount billed to insurance_____ Amount paid by insurance_____

Shortfall (difference between amount billed to insurance and the amount paid by insurance)

_____

Amount billed directly to patient_____ Amount paid by patient _____

Provider or product_____ Date_____

Copayment or amount paid toward deductible _____

Amount billed to insurance_____ Amount paid by insurance_____

Shortfall (difference between amount billed to insurance and the amount paid by insurance)

_____

Amount billed directly to patient_____ Amount paid by patient _____

Provider or product_____ Date_____

Copayment or amount paid toward deductible _____

Amount billed to insurance_____ Amount paid by insurance_____

Shortfall (difference between amount billed to insurance and the amount paid by insurance)

_____

Amount billed to insurance_____ Amount paid by insurance_____

FINANCIAL WORKSHEET: PART 1

Statement for (name) _____

Completed by _____

Date completed_____

For the month of _____

The purpose of this form is to make sure that the elderly person's average monthly expenses do not exceed his or her average monthly income. By completing this form as accurately as possible, you may discover problem areas that need to be adjusted in the future.

You will compare income and expenses over a time period of one month. It doesn't matter which month you choose. An elderly person's income and expenses shouldn't vary much from month to month, except in the case of a medical crisis, a change in living arrangements, the death of a spouse, or other such life change.

Before you begin, make several copies of the *Financial Worksheets.* Update the worksheets whenever there is a significant change in the elderly person's situation, and again compare income and expenses over a one-month period. With all your records on hand, including the completed *Vital Information Form,* you should be able to complete this worksheet within a few hours.

You will enter the cash available at the start of the month, the income received during the month, and the expenses paid during that month. For large receipts or payments that only occur at certain times of the year—such as a semiannual annuity payment or quarterly taxes—include an average monthly amount. For a semiannual tax payment, for example, you would enter one-sixth of the total semiannual payment, or one-twelfth of the annual; for a quarterly payment, you would enter one-fourth of the quarterly payment.

A Family Caregiver's Guide to Planning and Decision Making for the Elderly © 1999 James A. Wilkinson

CASH AND INCOME AVAILABLE AT THE BEGINNING OF THE MONTH

In the following section, record the cash and cash equivalents (such as food stamps) available at the beginning of the month. The column labeled "Partners" refers to accounts belonging to a spouse (or anyone who lives with the elderly person) whose funds are normally used to cover household expenses. If this person's funds are included in any of the other accounts, make sure you don't list them twice.

For each bank account, enter (1) the ending balance on the most recent monthly statement, depending on the month you're calculating and (2) the date of the statement. Note: The beginning and ending date of each statement may not be the same.

Because you're trying to measure the cash available for the month, if a month-end statement is unusually high or low, you can enter an average month-end balance instead. If the month-end checking account balance usually averages $300, but this month it is $800 because the rent check has not yet cleared the bank, it may be better to enter $300 instead of $800.

For brokerage and money market accounts, record only those balances that can be immediately converted to cash. Don't include stock or bond investments, which must be sold before they can be converted to cash.

	Elderly Person's	Partner's	Statement date
Cash on hand	_____	_____	N/A
Checking account	_____	_____	_____
Checking account	_____	_____	_____
Savings account	_____	_____	_____
Savings account	_____	_____	_____
Credit union	_____	_____	_____
Money market account	_____	_____	_____
Brokerage account	_____	_____	_____
Food stamps on hand	_____	_____	N/A
_____	_____	_____	_____
_____	_____	_____	_____
Total cash available	_____ +	_____ =	_____

INCOME RECEIVED OR EXPECTED FOR THE MONTH

Next, record income that will be available for use during the month. Record net income, that is, the amount left over after deductions. (Don't bother with totals under $10). For income received on a quarterly or semiannual basis, enter a monthly average. (Remember, you are trying to calculate average monthly income.) For example, if the elderly person receives a $2,100 semiannual annuity, the amount you list here is $350, or the semi-annual amount divided by 6.

Note: Make sure you don't count the same money twice by recording it both here and in a checking or savings account. If last month's total in the checking or savings account includes the $2,100 annuity payment, and you enter $350 in this section as well, you will have counted that annuity payment twice.

	Monthly amount	Date(s) received
Salary		
Partner's income		
Social Security		
Pension/Keogh		
Alimony		
Interest income		
Dividends		
IRA distributions		
Profit sharing		
Insurance proceeds		
Reverse mortgage		
Settlement payments (from a lawsuit, divorce, etc.)		
Annuity payments		
Trust distributions		
Note or loan income		
Cash from family members		
Rental income		

A Family Caregiver's Guide to Planning and Decision Making for the Elderly © 1999 James A. Wilkinson

Food stamps   _____   _____

Welfare/SSI   _____   _____

_____   _____   _____

_____   _____   _____

Total   _____   _____

TOTAL MONTHLY CASH AND INCOME

Add the amounts from the two previous sections to determine the person's available money for one month. Note: If your total doesn't seem like it's in the ballpark, you may have forgotten something or double-counted something. Check the *Vital Information Form* to be sure you have included all readily available cash and income.

Total cash and income available for the month _____

ROUTINE LIVING EXPENSES AND LIABILITIES

The next two tables list routine expenses incurred while living independently. If the need arises to explore other housing options, this information will help you compare the costs of alternative living arrangements.

The first table covers housing expenses. (Refer to the *Monthly Expense Forms* on pages 36 and 37 for much of the information you need.) If the cost for each service is not paid in full every month, enter the average monthly expense or budgeted payment. Some expenses, such as the cost of repairs, may be difficult to determine. Estimate, if necessary, considering the frequency and cost of past repairs, as well as the condition of the home, grounds, and appliances. Note: Services that are provided or paid for by family members—even if considered routine—should be included under Free Services on page 53.

The second table focuses on property taxes. If the elderly person has more than one residence, complete a separate chart for each residence. If the person rents, you probably won't need to complete this chart.

If more than one person lives in the household, but only one income is used, don't divide expenses. In the case of a dual-income household, you may want to use this information to calculate how the financial picture would change if one partner died or moved out. For example, if an elderly husband was admitted to a nursing home, his Social Security check would still come in, but much of it would likely be used to pay for his nursing home care, so less money would be available to cover household expenses.

1. Housing expenses (complete one for each residence)

	Account number	Balance/budget amount
Rent or mortgage payment		
Management/condo fees		
Property/renters insurance		
Repair and maintenance		
Telephone: local		
Telephone: long distance		
Electricity		
Cable/Satellite		
Water		
Sewer		
Garbage		
Gas or oil		

Lawn maintenance _____ _____

Snow removal _____ _____

Pool service _____ _____

Housecleaning _____ _____

Laundry/dry cleaning _____ _____

Newspaper or other subscriptions _____ _____

Security _____ _____

Geriatric care manager _____ _____

House sitter _____ _____

Pet sitter _____ _____

_____ _____ _____

2. Property taxes (complete one for each property owned)

	Date due	Average monthly amount
a. Residence		
State	_____	_____
County	_____	_____
Local	_____	_____
School	_____	_____
Personal property	_____	_____
Assessments	_____	_____
b. Additional property		
State	_____	_____
County	_____	_____
Local	_____	_____
School	_____	_____
Personal property	_____	_____
Assessments	_____	_____

3. Living expenses (not related to healthcare)

The *Monthly Expense Forms* on pages 36 and 37 allowed you to record individual transactions—every trip to the grocery store and every ride on the bus. Now, use the information on these forms to calculate monthly totals on the table that follows (the total amount spent on groceries, the total amount spent on bus transportation, and so forth). If you are completing this section without the help of the *Monthly Expense Forms,* try to estimate the totals.

Naturally, the information on the *Monthly Expense Forms* will change from month to month. However, the general trends should remain the same unless there has been a significant change in the elderly person's life (a medical crisis, a change in living arrangements, or the death of a spouse, for example). Therefore, if your records are good and there are no significant fluctuations from month to month, you may use the *Monthly Expense Forms* from any recent month when filling out this section.

Use the "comments" column to note the name of the payee, an unusual expense included, or your method of calculation—for example, if you divided last year's income taxes by 12.

	Average monthly amount	Comments
Federal, state, and local income taxes (based upon amounts paid last year)		
Groceries		
Dining out		
Personal items (alcohol, cigarettes)		
Transportation (taxis, bus, gasoline, automobile expenses)		
Entertainment (movies, bingo, golf fees, contests)		
Clothing		
Contributions (church, club dues)		
Beautician/barber		
Gifts and gratuities		
Insurance premiums other than property and health		
Miscellaneous expenses (see *Vital Information Form*)		

4. Healthcare expenses

Using the *Medical Charges and Payments Form* on page 38, enter an average monthly amount for each of the following categories (doctors, medications, and so forth). Include only out-of-pocket payments made by the elderly. Do not include charges paid by Medicare, Medicaid, or medical insurance unless you expect that these coverages will terminate in the near future and the services will need to continue at the elderly person's expense. Also, because net income is used in these worksheets, do not include payments that are automatically deducted from checks received, such as insurance premiums deducted from Social Security or pension checks.

	Average monthly amount	Comments
Medicare deductibles or copayments	_____	_____
Health insurance premiums	_____	_____
Other health insurance deductibles and copayments	_____	_____
Dentists	_____	_____
Doctors	_____	_____
Nurses	_____	_____
Therapists or psychologists	_____	_____
Medications	_____	_____
Medical device rentals (wheelchair, etc.)	_____	_____
Medical products and supplies (oxygen, IV, ostomy products, supplements)	_____	_____
Adult daycare or respite care services	_____	_____
Other home healthcare services	_____	_____
Share of Medicaid cost (portion of cost that is not paid by Medicaid)	_____	_____
_____	_____	_____
_____	_____	_____

5. Total living expenses

Add up the totals in sections 1 through 4. This should approximate the elderly person's total average monthly expenses. Compare this number with the total cash available for the month on page 42. If expenses are less than the income available, the elderly should not have to worry about their savings eroding, even if they must occasionally withdraw funds from their savings to meet unexpected expenses in a particular month.

Total expected expenses for the month _____

Now consider whether the difference between income and expenses reflects reality. If your calculations show more income than expenses, but in fact expenses have been higher than income for the last six months, something has been left out. If the discrepancy is significant, in either direction, recheck the worksheets.

You may find that even though the numbers are correct, expenses still appear smaller on paper than in reality. In this case, it's possible that the elderly person—or a relative with access to his or her accounts—has intentionally hidden certain expenses. In the case of deception or fraud, you may have to involve the police or postal inspectors. Most likely, a discrepancy is the result of poor record keeping or simply forgetting something. However, if a significant amount of money is missing, it's important to find out why.

FINANCIAL WORKSHEET: PART 2

Statement for (name)_____

Completed by _____

Date completed _____

The *Financial Worksheet: Part 1* assesses whether monthly cash flow is increasing or decreasing the elderly person's savings, and gives you a glimpse of whether the person can manage his or her own affairs. Part 2 helps to identify and categorize certain assets and liabilities to see if the elderly person's financial position can be strengthened, if assets need to be sold (and if so, which ones), and if there's a plan to meet the elderly person's future needs. Again, these worksheets will not tell you what to do or how to plan for future needs. They simply allow you to get a complete inventory before making such decisions. Unless you have a background in financial planning, it may be wise to seek the advice of a financial advisor, accountant, or attorney who works with the elderly.

Three notes of caution:

1. When deciding whether to sell assets, you'll need to know what each item is worth, how easily it can be sold, and what taxes (if any) will need to be paid. Remember, though, some items may have

been promised to someone else—an heir, for example. In such cases, serious family conflicts can arise when a caregiver sells or gives away possessions without the consent of the elderly person and other family members.

2. You cannot take, give away, or sell anything that is not yours, no matter how good your intentions. If you're not the elderly person's legal guardian, you must have his or her permission to dispose of his or her possessions, either directly or through a power of attorney. This is why it's essential to establish a durable power of attorney (see chapter 6) or legal guardianship before an emergency arises.

3. Caregivers should never confuse financial planning for the elderly with retirement planning for themselves. All too often, family members believe that once they begin providing caregiving services, they have the right to take or dispose of the elderly person's assets as they wish. Almost nothing could be worse than to endure the sacrifices required by caregiving and then face a legal challenge for theft.

ASSETS THAT COULD BE EASILY SOLD OR CONVERTED TO CASH

List all assets with an established market price. In other words, list those assets that can be easily sold, cashed in, or borrowed against.

The object of an investment is to wait until it matures or the price is right to sell. In an emergency, however, these investments are potential sources of cash. It's a good idea to determine which of these you would want to cash in first if a financial emergency should arise.

Asset	Estimated value
CDs (certificates of deposit)	_____
Savings bonds	_____
Publicly traded bonds	_____
Publicly traded notes	_____
Publicly traded stock	_____
Mutual fund shares	_____
IRA account value	_____
Keogh-type plan value	_____
401(k) plan value	_____
Life insurance (cash value)	_____
Life insurance (if the death benefit can be sold)	_____
_____	_____
_____	_____
_____	_____

ASSETS THAT COULD BE SOLD, BUT THE MARKET VALUE IS UNCERTAIN

Although the following assets could be sold, there's no way of knowing how long it would take or how much money you would get in return. Furthermore, selling any of these assets might lead to a change in lifestyle. The primary residence is a good example. Even if you know the house's approximate value, only by actually selling it would you know how much it would sell for, how quickly, and what the sale would cost in taxes, commissions, and psychological stress. You'd also need to decide where the elderly person would live after the house was sold and how much a new living arrangement would cost. (If the house is paid off, and you want to keep the house and increase monthly income, you might consider getting a "reverse mortgage," which pays a fixed monthly amount based on the value of the house.)

Be conservative when estimating the value of items listed under "Personal possessions." They will likely have a lower value than you think. If you are counting on selling these items to raise money in an emergency, get a firm bid from a dealer first. It's not foolproof, but it's better than relying on the item's original cost, a telephone quote, or the dollar value printed in a consumer's guide.

In an emergency, if items are in storage, on loan, or gathering dust in the attic, you could hold a garage sale or auction to raise cash. Stabilizing the elderly person's finances may be more important than the sentimental value attached to personal possessions or the family's desire to inherit these items.

Asset	Estimated value
Primary residence	_____
Secondary residence	_____
Condo/time share	_____
Automobile	_____
Automobile	_____
Rental property	_____
Undeveloped land	_____
Personal possessions	_____
_____	_____
_____	_____
_____	_____

ASSETS WITH LITTLE OR NO ESTABLISHED MARKET VALUE

To estimate the value of an asset that has no established market, remember that value is determined by what the item is worth to the buyer. Finding a buyer may be difficult because buyers have no guarantee that they'll be able to resell the item. Be very cautious in assessing estimated value here. Consider the uniqueness of the item, the potential market, the underlying value of the parts, and any restrictions on ownership.

Often, the item's original cost will have little to do with its current value. Consider a Christmas plate collection. Let's say the plates have been collected at $50 each over the last twenty years. The collection is probably worth less than its $1,000 cost, because most buyers are other plate collectors who already have these plates. However, if the $50 plates have been collected over forty years, there's a better chance that they're worth more than their $2,000 cost—the older plates may be hard to get, so collectors may pay quite a bit of money to fill out their own collection, even if they do not want or need most of the plates. Another example is privately held stock. Restrictions on transfer, rights of first refusal by other shareholders, or a fixed redemption price could limit value. Even without such legal barriers, finding a buyer may be difficult, giving that buyer substantial leverage in negotiating the sale price.

Asset	Estimated value
Private stock	_____
Unsecured loans	_____
Collections	_____
Personal possessions	_____
_____	_____
_____	_____
_____	_____

A Family Caregiver's Guide to Planning and Decision Making for the Elderly © 1999 James A. Wilkinson

LARGE LIABILITIES

Up to this point, your main concern has been making sure that the elderly person has enough money to cover routine expenses, hopefully without having to sell off assets. In this section, you will determine how large expenses and liabilities affect the elderly person's overall financial situation. By knowing that large liabilities exist, you may be able to help the elderly person plan his or her finances accordingly—namely, whether to set aside enough money to pay off these liabilities or take steps to eliminate them.

You will also look for potential liabilities. For example, if you think you might need to make a large deposit to get into a particular assisted-living facility in the future, note this in the table. This is a potential liability, and you should plan where this money would come from.

Reducing debts and eliminating liabilities may improve the elderly person's financial position and reduce his or her psychological stress. However, if you do not consider all the ramifications, the consequences could be significant. In an emergency, a professional might be able to suggest options you hadn't considered that would allow the elderly person to raise cash without eliminating liabilities, such as arranging a reverse mortgage or collecting on a life insurance policy before death.

Type	Estimated amount
Mortgage	_____
Federal taxes due this year	_____
State taxes due this year	_____
Local taxes due this year	_____
Estimated estate taxes (if funds are not available when one spouse dies)	_____
Known major repairs or expenses	_____
Anticipated housing deposits (for a nursing home or assisted living facility, for example)	_____
Existing personal loans	_____
Existing unreimbursed medical expenses	_____
_____	_____
_____	_____

FREE SERVICES AND SIGNIFICANTLY DISCOUNTED EXPENSES

In this section, record any free or discounted products and services that the elderly person receives. Also note who provides these products and services and how much money is saved.

"Free" means free to the elderly person—even if the item or service is donated or provided at a cost to someone else (such as free room and board or gifts of food, clothing, travel, home repair or maintenance). A significantly discounted expense might come through a special program, such as a gas subsidy for seniors. Don't include senior discounts on movie tickets or dining—the elderly person may give up going to movies and eating out in the future; he or she might also start going to theaters or restaurants where these discounts don't apply.

The idea here is to (1) list any products or services that might create financial problems if the elderly person suddenly had to pay for them, and (2) think of ways to replace these products and services if they are taken away. For example, if the bus company decides they will no longer offer free rides to seniors, the elderly person would have to pay to ride the bus. However, if bus service was canceled or if the person's physical condition deteriorated, the next option might be to take a taxi.

Most caregivers donate substantial amounts of their own money to their elderly charge's care. If you are a caregiver, this section can help you determine what you are really spending, how long you can afford to help, and what support you need from others. You can also note any services that might have to be replaced in the future, even if the cost is insignificant. For example, if someone from church takes the elderly person to the hairdresser every week, it's helpful to think about how you would replace that service if it were no longer available.

1. Free goods or services

Goods or services	Provider	Estimated monthly savings

2. Significantly discounted expenses

Expense	Provider	Estimated monthly savings
_____	_____	_____
_____	_____	_____
_____	_____	_____
_____	_____	_____
_____	_____	_____

Chapter 3

Collecting Medical Information

This chapter is designed to do three things:

1. Provide healthcare professionals with basic medical information in an emergency, either because the elderly person is unable to provide the information or because his or her medical records aren't immediately available.

2. Help the elderly person and caregivers manage medications being taken.

3. Record the caregiver's observations about how the elderly person manages certain daily activities.

The forms in this chapter are not intended for diagnosis or treatment, nor are they a substitute for official medical records. However, they should be completed, updated periodically, and kept handy in case of emergency. Some forms may also be useful to alternative caregivers, who may not know the elderly person's medical history and medication needs.

This chapter contains six forms:

1. *Basic Medical Information* (page 57), a listing of names and phone numbers of doctors, hospitals, and insurers who have the elderly person's medical records. This form should be carried by the elderly person at all times.

2. *Medical History* (page 62), a summary of the person's medical history and information about his or her direct family members. This form should be carried by the elderly person at all times.

3. *Medication List* (page 70), a list of all medications (both prescribed and over-the-counter) the person is taking, instructions for each medication, and other essential information.

4. *Medication Summary* (page 73), a summary of the medications listed on the *Medication List*. This form should be carried by the elderly person at all times.

5. *Medication Schedule* (page 74), a daily schedule to help patients and caregivers remember when each medicine is to be taken, and how much to take.

6. *Activities of Daily Living Checklist* (page 77), an assessment of the elderly person's ability to perform everyday activities.

As you may have noticed, several of these forms should be carried by the elderly person at all times. Copies of these should also be given to family members and friends who might be contacted in an emergency (if the elderly person cannot provide medical information because he or she is unconscious or confused).

All forms in this chapter must be updated periodically to ensure that the information is accurate.

Always date each form as it is revised. Remember, these forms are not a substitute for medical records, but if properly completed, they can direct health professionals to information they need, including official records.

As you gather medical information, be aware that the elderly may not want to disclose certain matters, especially to you. While being generally truthful, they may withhold specific information or attempt to please doctors or family members by telling them what they want to hear. Some elderly people may not admit that they've been to see an acupuncturist, chiropractor, or naturopath, for instance; others may minimize alcohol or tobacco consumption, or fail to disclose an unbalanced diet. In some cases, an elderly person might cover up a spouse's mental or physical problems, fearing that the family or doctor will want to institutionalize him or her.

Try to help the elderly understand that full disclosure is the best policy. Explain that doctors need complete and accurate information in order to treat the problem correctly, and early treatment may prevent the condition from getting worse.

Documenting Medical History

What You Need to Know

If you were called in the middle of the night by an emergency room nurse who said your father-in-law had had an apparent heart attack, would you know his primary care doctor or recent medical history? Having this information may save the emergency room staff critical time in obtaining medical records—it could even save a life. It's important for every elderly person, caregiver, and family member to have a copy of the person's *Basic Medical Information* and *Medical History*. They should also be able to tell healthcare workers where to find original medical records.

The elderly person should carry his or her medical history at all times. For certain conditions, a medical identification bracelet may be a good idea in the event of an emergency. You can discuss this with the elderly person and his or her doctor.

How to Use the *Basic Medical Information* and *Medical History* Forms

These forms will help you collect essential information about the elderly person's medical history. While they cannot be used in place of official medical records, they will explain where these records are located and, to some extent, what they contain.

The *Medical History* form, in particular, should focus on the most recent medical events, conditions, and treatments. Recent events are more valuable in assessing the person's current medical condition and are more likely to be accurate and verifiable. Any information given from memory that can't be confirmed by the person's primary doctor should be treated with caution.

BASIC MEDICAL INFORMATION

Along with the *Medication List* on page 70, this is one of the most important forms to keep updated, especially when the primary doctor changes or hospitalization occurs. If you need more room to list all of the relevant information, add another page and staple it to this form.

In a medical emergency, the doctor can use this information to quickly locate the patient's medical records. When time is critical, the information here (and on the *Medication List*) can be a starting point for treatment. Furthermore, section 8 will alert a doctor if someone has been designated to provide informed consent for treatment.

This form should be carried with the elderly person at all times, especially when traveling.

This form completed by (circle one) patient • caregiver

Date completed _____

Copy given to _____

Telephone number _____

Copy given to _____

Telephone number _____

1. Patient information

Patient name _____

Patient address _____

_____

Patient home telephone number _____

The patient is: single • married • widowed • divorced • separated

Patient Social Security number _____

Patient blood type _____

Patient date and place of birth

_____

2. Primary care information

List current primary doctor, medical practice group, or clinic where recent medical records are most likely available.

Name _____

Address _____

_____

Telephone number _____

3. Specialists seen in the last two years

Name _____

Specialty _____

Address _____

Telephone number _____

Name _____

Specialty _____

Address _____

Telephone number _____

4. Hospital admissions in the last three years

Hospital _____

Date/reason for admission _____

Address _____

_____

Telephone number _____

Hospital _____

Date/reason for admission _____

Address _____

_____

Telephone number _____

5. Other medical treatments in the last three years

List nursing home, rehabilitation hospital, home healthcare agency, acupuncturist, chiropractor, naturopath, and so forth.

Provider name_____

Address _____

_____

Telephone number _____

Provider name_____

Address _____

_____

Telephone number _____

6. Pharmacy where most prescriptions are filled

Name of pharmacy _____

Address _____

Telephone number _____

7. Laboratory work (MRI, CT scans, cardiac catheterization)

Name of laboratory _____

Address _____

Telephone number _____

8. Insurance and legal information

a. Does the patient have a durable healthcare power of attorney?   yes • no

If yes, where is the original? _____

b. Does the patient have a living will?   yes • no

If yes, where is the original? _____

c. Primary health insurance provider or Medicare claim information

Copy both sides of insurance card and staple to back of page.

Provider name_____

Patient, member, or Medicare claim number _____

Group number _____

If insured through employer, employer's name and address

_____

_____

Prenotification telephone number _____

d. Supplemental or Medigap health insurance provider

Copy both sides of insurance card and staple to back of page.

Provider name_____

Patient or member number_____

Contract and/or group number_____

If insured through employer, employer's name and address

_____

_____

Prenotification telephone number _____

e. Other health insurance information or prenotification requirements

_____

_____

_____

_____

_____

_____

_____

MEDICAL HISTORY

This form completed by (circle one) patient • caregiver

Date completed _____

Patient name _____

Patient address _____

_____

Patient home telephone number _____

The patient is: single • married • widowed • divorced • separated

Patient Social Security number _____

Patient date and place of birth _____

1. Has the patient ever been treated for any of the following conditions?

Check all conditions that apply, providing information related to ongoing treatment or medication for the condition. If necessary, continue on back of page.

[ ] AIDS _____

[ ] Anemia _____

[ ] Aneurysm _____

[ ] Arthritis _____

[ ] Asthma/lung problems _____

[ ] Blood pressure (high or low) _____

[ ] Bowel problems _____

[ ] Cancer _____

[ ] Chest pain _____

[ ] Dementia _____

[ ] Diabetes _____

[ ] Eczema _____

[ ] Epilepsy/seizures _____

[ ] Eye problems _____

[ ] Gout _____

[ ] Heart disease _____

[ ] Herpes/gonorrhea _____

[ ] Kidney/bladder disease _____

[ ] Liver/gallbladder disease _____

[ ] Mental illness _____

[ ] Migraines _____

[ ] Orthopedic surgery _____

[ ] Osteoarthritis _____

[ ] Osteoporosis _____

[ ] Phlebitis _____

[ ] Sciatica _____

[ ] Skin disease _____

[ ] Stroke _____

[ ] Swallowing problems _____

[ ] Thyroid disorders _____

[ ] Ulcers/colitis _____

[ ] Urinary problems _____

Please describe other known medical conditions not listed.

_____

_____

Does the patient use corrective lenses, a hearing aid, or any assistive devices?

_____

_____

2. Has the patient been hospitalized within the last year?

yes • no

If "yes," was surgery involved? Is the patient still receiving treatment or taking medication? (List below)

Date of hospitalization _____ Surgery _____

Ongoing treatment/medication _____

_____

_____

3. Is the patient allergic to any medications?

_____

_____

4. Does the patient have an advance directive (durable healthcare power of attorney, living will)?

_____

_____

If applicable, who has the original?

Name _____

Phone number _____

5. Has the patient ever lived in a residential facility, such as a nursing home, where medical care was provided?

Name/type of facility _____ Time period _____

Reason for leaving _____

_____

_____

6. The following is known about the patient's family medical history:

a. Mother

Born (date) _____ Died (date)_____ Age_____

Cause of death _____

Known medical conditions _____

_____

_____

b. Maternal grandmother

Born (date) _____ Died (date)_____ Age_____

Cause of death _____

Known medical conditions _____

_____

_____

c. Maternal grandfather

Born (date) _____ Died (date)_____ Age_____

Cause of death _____

Known medical conditions _____

_____

_____

d. Father

Born (date) _____ Died (date)_____ Age_____

Cause of death _____

Known medical conditions _____

_____

_____

e. Paternal grandmother

Born (date) _____ Died (date)_____ Age_____

Cause of death _____

Known medical conditions _____

_____

_____

f. Paternal grandfather

Born (date) _____ Died (date)_____ Age_____

Cause of death _____

Known medical conditions _____

_____

_____

g. Brother or sister (circle one)

Born (date) _____ Died (date)_____ Age_____

Cause of death _____

Known medical conditions _____

_____

_____

Brother or sister (circle one)

Born (date) _____ Died (date)_____ Age_____

Cause of death _____

Known medical conditions _____

_____

_____

Brother or sister (circle one)

Born (date) _____ Died (date)_____ Age_____

Cause of death _____

Known medical conditions _____

_____

_____

h. Children: male or female (circle one)

Born (date) _____ Died (date)_____ Age_____

Cause of death _____

Known medical conditions _____

_____

_____

Children: male or female (circle one)

Born (date) _____ Died (date)_____ Age_____

Cause of death _____

Known medical conditions _____

_____

_____

Children: male or female (circle one)

Born (date) _____ Died (date)_____ Age_____

Cause of death _____

Known medical conditions _____

_____

_____

.

i. Other family member

Relationship _____

Born (date) _____ Died (date)_____ Age_____

Cause of death _____

Known medical conditions _____

_____

_____

Other family member

Relationship _____

Born (date) _____ Died (date)_____ Age_____

Cause of death _____

Known medical conditions _____

_____

_____

Other family member

Relationship _____

Born (date) _____ Died (date)_____ Age_____

Cause of death _____

Known medical conditions _____

_____

_____

Keeping Track of Medications

What You Need to Know

The consumption of medications—both prescribed and over-the-counter—is one of the most serious issues facing the elderly today. Even life-saving medications can become life-threatening when overused, misused, or abused. Also, the way the aging body absorbs and processes medications is not well understood, and the likelihood of adverse reactions increases with the number of medications a person is taking.

Usage Guidelines

The elderly and their caregivers can minimize adverse reactions by taking certain common-sense precautions:

1. Follow the doctor's exact instructions regarding what time to take the prescription, what to take it with (food or water, for example), and how long to take it.

2. The elderly should never stop a medication without telling their doctor, even if the medication does not appear to be working or if an over-the-counter alternative is cheaper. The medicine was prescribed for a reason.

3. If taking a prescription medication, the elderly should never start taking another medication—even an over-the-counter supplement—without consulting their doctor.

4. Find out everything you can about each prescribed drug in order to monitor its effectiveness and recognize problems. The elderly and their caregivers should know what each drug is supposed to do, how it works, how it should be taken, the length of time it must be taken, how it reacts with other drugs, what its potential side effects are, and if alternative medications are available. Use the *Medication List* on page 70 to discuss these issues with the doctor(s) involved.

5. The elderly should not, under any circumstances, trade medications with their friends.

6. Elderly patients and their caregivers should be absolutely candid with doctors and pharmacists about diet, prescription drugs, over-the-counter medications, and accuracy in complying with prescriptions. Eating poorly or failing to take prescriptions according to instructions can affect the way the body absorbs and processes drugs.

7. If you suspect an adverse drug reaction and the doctor doesn't seem concerned, get a second opinion. When in doubt, contact the prescribing doctor first. If you're not satisfied with the explanation or if you remain concerned, seek a second opinion from another doctor or pharmacist.

8. With any new drug, if the patient suddenly experiences problems with balance, vision, hearing, mental capacity, verbal coherence, or even emotional stability, contact the doctor immediately.

9. Get into the habit of asking the following questions about any new prescription:
   - What will this medication do?
   - What are the expected side effects?
   - How can the side effects be relieved?
   - How long should this medicine be taken?
   - Is there an alternative therapy that does not require medication?
   - What happens if a dose is missed?
   - Is this medicine habit-forming?
   - After reviewing the *Medication List,* do you see any possible adverse drug interactions?

10. Tell the doctor about any alcohol intake, even if it's minimal, before starting new medications. The *Medication List* purposely excludes alcohol and recreational drugs. Although the use of recreational drugs isn't common among the elderly, use of alcohol is. Alcohol consumption must be mentioned to the doctor or pharmacist,

especially if it's habitual—a few drinks each day or several drinks on social occasions. A depressant, alcohol causes adverse reactions with many medications. This is especially important if the elderly person drives—when alcohol combines with certain medications, it can affect alertness and reaction time.

11. Don't forget to tell the doctor about use of laxatives, vitamins, herbs, and supplements. Many elderly people take large doses of vitamins, supplements, and herbs. Space is provided to list these on the *Medication List*. If supplements are being taken, the doctor needs to know so he or she can determine possible drug interactions.

12. Tell the doctor about any allergic reactions, digestive problems, breathing problems, or emotional effects caused by previous medications.

Pharmacists

While the patient may have several doctors, it is seldom wise to have more than one pharmacist. For chronic conditions, an elderly person may use a mail-order company, such as AARP's Pharmacy Service, to minimize costs or comply with insurance requirements. However, the person should use only one local pharmacist to fill prescriptions. Take advantage of the pharmacist's expertise and services, including delivery, large print labels, ID bracelets, and the monitoring of prescriptions. Pharmacists are a key resource; do not hesitate to use them, especially to answer questions about a new prescription and possible drug interactions.

How to Use the Medication Forms

The following section contains the *Medication List*, the *Medication Summary*, and the *Medication Schedule* for people who take medications at different times of the day. The most important form is the *Medication List*, which records key information about all drugs and medications being taken.

Keeping Forms Up-to-Date

Up-to-date information about the medications a person is taking is important for many reasons. If a prescription is lost, but you have the prescription number and the name of the pharmacy, you may save yourself a visit to the doctor or clinic to get a new prescription. Up-do-date information will also help your doctor identify unnecessary or inappropriate medications. Finally, when the patient's circumstances change, up-to-date information will help the doctor know when a medication should be reduced, increased, or discontinued.

The *Medication List* should be reviewed by a doctor before any new drug is introduced. If the doctor can see a list of every product that is being taken, used, or applied, the possibility of drug-related medical problems decreases.

Cleaning Out the Medicine Cabinet

As you fill out the medication forms, discard all expired or unused pills, ointments, and liquids, including both prescription and over-the-counter products such as laxatives, vitamins, and cold remedies. Also, make sure that prescriptions have not been randomly mixed, that they are stored properly, that the lid is fastened, and that they are being taken as directed.

Elderly people often leave medications open, mix them with other medications, or don't take them at all because they find it difficult to open the container. Once medications are mixed, there's no way to tell how old they are or why they are being taken. If you run across a medication you're unsure about, ask your pharmacist for help, or discard it.

MEDICATION LIST

The *Medication List* will be your main source of information for filling out the following medication forms. It should be updated as medications change. On this form, you will:

1. List all the drugs and medications the elderly person is taking.
2. Provide specific information about each medication.
3. Explain why each medication is being taken.

Generally, the information you need to fill out this form will be on the label of the prescription or over-the-counter product. All prescriptions should be listed, even if some are only taken as needed. Include medications taken internally by mouth or nose, or via a patch, suppository, or injection, as well as those applied externally to the skin, ears, or eyes. With over-the-counter products such as aspirin, herbs, vitamins, or laxatives, list only those taken routinely by mouth or applied to the skin or eyes.

Patient name _____

Date completed_____ Completed by_____

Date updated_____ Updated by_____

Known drug allergies/reactions

_____

_____

PRESCRIPTION MEDICATIONS

1. Prescription number _____

Doctor_____

Medication _____

Generic name _____

Instructions _____

Purpose _____

Dosage _____

Color/description _____

Pharmacy _____

Mail order_____

Date prescribed_____ Expiration date_____

Refills _____

2. Prescription number _____

Doctor_____

Medication _____

Generic name _____

Instructions _____

Purpose _____

Dosage _____

Color/description _____

Pharmacy _____

Mail order_____

Date prescribed_____ Expiration date_____

Refills _____

3. Prescription number _____

Doctor_____

Medication _____

Generic name _____

Instructions _____

Purpose _____

Dosage _____

Color/description _____

Pharmacy _____

Mail order _____

Date prescribed_____ Expiration date_____

Refills _____

4. Prescription number _____

Doctor_____

Medication _____

Generic name _____

Instructions _____

Purpose _____

Dosage _____

Color/description _____

Pharmacy _____

Mail order _____

Date prescribed_____ Expiration date_____

Refills _____

5. Prescription number _____

Doctor_____

Medication _____

Generic name _____

Instructions _____

Purpose _____

Dosage _____

Color/description _____

Pharmacy _____

Mail order _____

Date prescribed_____ Expiration date_____

Refills _____

6. Prescription number

Doctor_____

Medication _____

Generic name _____

Instructions _____

Purpose _____

Dosage _____

Color/description _____

Pharmacy _____

Mail order _____

Date prescribed_____ Expiration date_____

Refills _____

OTHER MEDICATIONS AND PRODUCTS

1. Name of medication/product/ supplement

_____

When taken (daily, as needed, and so forth)

_____

Dosage (size) _____

Color/description _____

2. Name of medication/product/ supplement

_____

When taken (daily, as needed, and so forth)

_____

Dosage (size) _____

Color/description _____

3. Name of medication/product/ supplement

_____

When taken (daily, as needed, and so forth)

_____

Dosage (size) _____

Color/description _____

4. Name of medication/product/ supplement

_____

When taken (daily, as needed, and so forth)

_____

Dosage (size) _____

Color/description _____

5. Name of medication/product/ supplement

_____

When taken (daily, as needed, and so forth)

_____

Dosage (size) _____

Color/description _____

6. Name of medication/product/ supplement

_____

When taken (daily, as needed, and so forth)

_____

Dosage (size) _____

Color/description _____

MEDICATION SUMMARY

Patient name _____

Date completed_____ Completed by _____

Known drug allergies/reactions

_____

_____

The patient should always carry a copy of this form. One of the first questions emergency room staff ask is, "What medications are you taking?" This form will show them all the medications the patient is using.

It's important to keep the *Medication Summary* up-to-date. This should be easy to do, because all the information comes from the *Medication List* on page 70. Take a few minutes to update this form whenever a medication is added or deleted, or a dosage is changed.

Medication/product	Purpose	Dosage	Instructions
_____	_____	_____	_____
_____	_____	_____	_____
_____	_____	_____	_____
_____	_____	_____	_____
_____	_____	_____	_____
_____	_____	_____	_____
_____	_____	_____	_____
_____	_____	_____	_____
_____	_____	_____	_____
_____	_____	_____	_____
_____	_____	_____	_____
_____	_____	_____	_____
_____	_____	_____	_____
_____	_____	_____	_____
_____	_____	_____	_____

MEDICATION SCHEDULE

This schedule is a list of times medicines are to be taken throughout the day. It should include the name of each medication, dosage, and any special instructions (such as "take with milk"). This will help an elderly person who occasionally gets confused about when to take his or her pills, as well as a temporary caregiver who isn't familiar with the elderly person's routine.

The *Medication Schedule* can be used over and over again until a prescription changes, or a new copy can be used each day so the elderly person can cross out a medication after taking it. Some caregivers premix medications in plastic bags and staple these to the appropriate time slots on the schedule. The elderly person can simply remove the bags and take the medications at the correct times. (If a new schedule is used each day, be sure to fill in the "date" line at the top.)

If the elderly person takes a number of medications or occasionally is confused about when to take them, caregivers can code the labels on the prescriptions with a sticker or magic marker—yellow for morning, red for evening, and so on. Another method is to mark each prescription label with a colored slash that correlates with a colored slash on the *Medication Schedule.* Yet another option is to mix pills in colored containers. No matter what the system, make sure that the elderly person fully understands it. Record the system on page 75 as a reminder.

Note: While this form can serve as a memory aid for caregivers, do not use any kind of unsupervised system if the elderly person has short-term memory loss or dementia, or is not capable of taking medication safely according to directions.

Patient _____

Date _____

Before breakfast

_____

_____

_____

_____

Breakfast

_____

_____

_____

_____

Lunch

_____

_____

_____

_____

Dinner

_____

_____

_____

_____

After dinner

_____

_____

_____

_____

At bedtime

_____

_____

_____

_____

COLOR CODE

Below, list the times of day that medications are to be taken, then list the corresponding colors used on prescription labels that represent these times of the day.

Time of day   Color

_____   _____

_____   _____

_____   _____

_____   _____

_____   _____

_____   _____

_____   _____

_____   _____

_____   _____

_____   _____

_____   _____

_____   _____

_____   _____

_____   _____

Activities of Daily Living

What You Need to Know

When a child says, "I have a pain in my leg," he or she most likely has a problem in the leg. But with the elderly, there's often no apparent connection between the location of the symptom and the location of the problem, so diagnosing and assessing the severity of the problem can be particularly difficult, even for an experienced clinician.

While it's difficult to link a physical symptom to a precise condition, the sudden inability to perform a common activity is something caregivers should take seriously. This is often the first sign of disease or illness. The early treatment of conditions that disrupt daily activities is critical to maintaining the elderly person's quality of life. According to Dr. Richard Besdine, author of *Evaluating the Elderly Patient: The Case for Assessment Technology,* disease can affect an elderly person's ability to function in several ways, including:

- The loss of desire to eat or drink
- A tendency to fall
- Incontinence or constipation
- Dizziness or lightheadedness
- Sudden confusion
- The onset or worsening of mild dementia
- Sudden weight loss
- A failure to thrive (the person's condition deteriorates despite proper eating, sleeping, exercise, and so forth)

The Merck Manual of Geriatrics summarizes these points: "The reasons that disease in the elderly manifests itself first as functional loss, often in organ systems unrelated to the [location] of illness, are not well understood.... Deterioration of functional independence in active, previously unimpaired elders is an early, subtle sign of untreated illness, usually without the typical symptoms and signs of the disease."

How to Use the *Activities of Daily Living Checklist*

On the checklist that follows, you will collect information about the elderly person's ability to perform routine activities. You can then present this information to a doctor or therapist. The picture you provide of the elderly person's ability to function is a vital part of a comprehensive geriatric assessment and a complete medical history.

Researchers have developed various methods for measuring the abilities necessary for independent living, including two classifications often used by professionals: Activities of Daily Living (ADLs) and Intermediate Activities of Daily Living (IADLs). ADLs primarily measure physical abilities, while IADLs attempt to measure social skills—the ability to plan, reason, and act.

A final classification, Advanced Activities of Daily Living (AADLs), is not discussed in this book. These are complex activities such as playing bridge, doing crossword puzzles, planning a party, or jogging. An elderly person who is capable of performing these activities will have little need for daily care. Ceasing to perform AADLs may be strictly voluntary. Ceasing to perform ADLs and IADLs, on the other hand, is seldom voluntary and generally reflects an underlying medical problem.

There is no scoring system on this checklist. The intent is not to diagnose, but rather to be able to report observations to a medical professional. However, if the elderly person is unable to function in several areas or routinely needs major assistance in even one ADL category, medical advice or a comprehensive geriatric assessment may be warranted.

ACTIVITIES OF DAILY LIVING CHECKLIST

Patient name_____

Date completed_____ Completed by _____

While few of these scenarios will fit your situation exactly, you can help a professional focus on potential problem areas by selecting the best answers to the following questions. The answers may also help identify a need for specific caregiving services and determine if the current caregiving arrangement is adequate.

ACTIVITIES OF DAILY LIVING

This first list focuses on the most basic activities of daily living, or ADLs, measuring the elderly person's ability to perform them without assistance. A mental or physical disability can lead to difficulty in any of these areas. The inability to perform even one of these activities is serious and will require caregiving assistance. For each of the following activities, check the level of assistance the elderly person requires.

Bathing
[ ] No assistance needed
[ ] Can bathe, but is often dirty
[ ] Some help needed
[ ] Lacks strength or agility to bathe safely

Continence
[ ] Full control of bladder and bowels
[ ] Occasional bladder accidents
[ ] Occasional bowel accidents
[ ] Accidents caused by decreased mental capacity
[ ] Regular problems with bladder or bowels— needs diaper

Dressing
[ ] No assistance needed
[ ] May need help with certain things, such as buttons or shoes

[ ] Can dress if someone selects clothes
[ ] Can dress, but isn't concerned about clothes or appearance
[ ] Needs help dressing and undressing

Eating
[ ] No assistance needed
[ ] Needs some help
[ ] Forgets to eat or eats at odd times
[ ] Can feed self, but needs help with certain foods or a specific diet
[ ] Swallowing problems; food must be pureed
[ ] Must be fed

Moving around
[ ] No assistance needed
[ ] Needs walker/cane for balance or support
[ ] Needs to hold onto someone or something
[ ] Needs wheelchair
[ ] Can move around, but waits for assistance
[ ] Needs help getting in or out of chairs
[ ] Needs help getting in or out of bed
[ ] Essentially bedridden

Using toilet
[ ] No assistance needed
[ ] Needs assistance getting on or off toilet
[ ] Needs assistance getting clothes off or on
[ ] Forgets what the toilet is for
[ ] Needs bedpan or portable toilet at night
[ ] Needs bedpan or portable toilet both day and night

A Family Caregiver's Guide to Planning and Decision Making for the Elderly © 1999 James A. Wilkinson

INTERMEDIATE ACTIVITIES OF DAILY LIVING

This list covers what are considered intermediate activities, or IADLs—a person's ability to complete tasks that require simple planning, reasoning, and judgment. Although some of these topics may raise gender issues (an elderly man may never have prepared his own meals, for example), try to determine if the person would be able to perform the task.

Housework

[ ] Knows what needs to be done and does it without prompting
[ ] Will do it, but only if prompted
[ ] Cannot do it, even if prompted

Taking medicine

[ ] Remembers to take medicine according to directions
[ ] Will take it according to directions if reminded
[ ] Cannot be trusted to take medicine properly, even if reminded

Preparing meals

[ ] Can plan and prepare a meal
[ ] Cannot plan, but can prepare a simple meal if assisted
[ ] Cannot plan or prepare even a simple meal

Managing money

[ ] Can manage finances and pay bills
[ ] Cannot manage finances, but can write checks with help
[ ] Cannot manage finances or pay bills

Minor repairs

[ ] Can identify problem and either fix it or call for assistance
[ ] Knows something is wrong, but cannot fix even simple things
[ ] Cannot identify problem, not even to ask for assistance

Telephone

[ ] Can use the telephone and find a number
[ ] Can use the telephone if number is known
[ ] Cannot use the telephone

Traveling

[ ] Can travel alone using private or public transportation
[ ] Can plan travel, but needs assistance
[ ] Can travel beyond neighborhood only if all arrangements have been made
[ ] Cannot travel alone under any circumstances

Chapter 4

Caring for the Elderly at Home

Most elderly people prefer to live at home for as long as possible, and most caregivers will do everything they can to help them maintain their independence. But as an elderly person's condition deteriorates, it may no longer be safe to live at home without assistance. It is the caregiver's job to determine how much assistance the elderly person needs, and whether a new living arrangement is necessary.

This chapter offers guidelines for helping the elderly live safely in their home for as long as possible. It covers long-distance caregiving, home safety, assistive devices, and how to hire home healthcare, housekeeping, and home maintenance services. The next chapter addresses issues that arise when living at home is simply no longer appropriate.

Making a Home Safe for the Elderly

What You Need to Know

Just as parents would inspect their home for anything that could injure a toddler, it's important for caregivers to evaluate the home for things that could injure an elderly person. The *Home Safety Checklists* that follow will help you make the elderly person's home safe, secure, and "elder-friendly," without spending too much money or making the living area look like a hospital or nursing home.

Throughout this chapter, the word "home" means any place the elderly person lives or spends time, whether a house, apartment, trailer, or condominium. If the elderly spend time in more than one home, each location should be evaluated. For example, if an elderly mother lives with her daughter but also spends time at her son's home, both houses should be reviewed for safety.

If you're not sure that it's safe for an elderly person to live alone without caregiving support, read Assessing the Risk of Living at Home on page 96.

How to Use the *Home Safety Checklists*

The checklists that follow will alert you to potential problems and difficulties that the average household can pose for an elderly person. Once you are aware of a problem, in most cases, you can take steps to keep accidents from happening. The checklists are organized by floor (basement, first floor, second floor), but some safety issues are room specific.

The *Home Safety Checklists* are designed to accommodate the average elderly person. If the person has a severe heart condition, or poor eyesight or hearing, additional precautions will need to be taken. If you're not aware of the adjustments necessary to accommodate a particular physical or emotional disability, seek professional advice, particularly from some of the organizations listed in chapter 7.

As you go through the *Home Safety Checklists,* don't assume that you or the elderly person must pay for all the repairs and modifications personally. Doctor-prescribed medical equipment and assistive devices may be covered by Medicare or Medicaid (as discussed on page 100), and other federal and state programs can provide financial assistance as well. For example, the Farmers Home Administration provides loans and grants for rural low-income elderly people. Other federal programs include the Department of Energy's Low-Income Home Energy Assistance Program (LIHEAP) and the Weatherization Assistance Program (WAP). Some cities, too, have special programs or will make community development block grant funds available to help senior citizens upgrade and maintain their homes. To find out more, check with your local Area Agency on Aging.

HOME SAFETY CHECKLISTS

LIGHTING AND ELECTRICAL SAFETY

Poor lighting is the most common reason that elderly people fall. While some accidents are caused by weak vision or not paying attention, most occur because the lighting is poor and the person cannot see properly. The following safety issues should be considered:

1. Rooms should be uniformly lit, without dark areas.

2. Light bulbs should be 75 to 100 watts.

3. Light switches should contrast with the color of the wall. They should be located just inside the door of each room and at the top and bottom of any stairs. If the room's light is not hooked up to a light switch, the path from the door to the lamp or other light fixture should be unobstructed and at least partly lit by light from another room.

4. Avoid backlighting and indirect lighting, especially if they create glare. Likewise, blinding glare from sunlight should be blocked with window blinds or curtains.

5. Install electric timers on lights to keep hallways and passages well lit at night. Lighting the path from the bedroom to the bathroom with night lights is a good idea, too.

6. Outdoor lights, located on the porch, driveway, stairway, or hallway, should provide enough light so the elderly can not only approach and leave the home safely, but also identify anyone approaching or standing at the door at night.

7. In heavily traveled areas and near stairs, replace wall light switches with large levers, especially if the switch is in an awkward place.

8. If the elderly have difficulty grasping or turning small objects, replace the twist knobs on lamp switches with push-bar switches.

9. Schedule routine light bulb changes, especially for hard-to-reach sockets. This minimizes the chance that a burned-out bulb will cause an accident because of inadequate lighting or because the elderly person tries to change it alone.

10. Make sure all electrical cords are in good condition (no bare wires) and tucked out of the way.

11. If the home has only two-prong outlets, keep three-prong adapters handy. Many appliances have a three-prong plug.

12. Make sure that outlets and extension cords are not overloaded.

13. Keep flashlights on hand for power outages. Flashlights are easier and safer to use than candles. Have several flashlights available and easily accessible throughout the house. For emergencies, attach a whistle to the flashlight clip (especially the one in the bedroom).

Lighting and Electrical Checklist

	Basement	First floor	Second floor
Uniformly lighted?	_____	_____	_____
Adequate wattage?	_____	_____	_____
Light switches: type, size, location?	_____	_____	_____
Pathway clear?	_____	_____	_____
No glare?	_____	_____	_____
Timers?	_____	_____	_____
Night lights needed?	_____	_____	_____
Adequate outdoor lighting?	_____	_____	_____
Replace lamp switches with push bars?	_____	_____	_____
Light bulb replacement plan?	_____	_____	_____
Cords out of the way?	_____	_____	_____
Three-prong adapters?	_____	_____	_____
No overloaded outlets?	_____	_____	_____
Flashlights accessible?	_____	_____	_____

RUG, CARPET, AND STAIR SAFETY

1. Repair, remove, or replace worn, threadbare, or torn rugs and carpets.

2. Look for abrupt changes in the walking surface (such as from a smooth wood floor to a thick carpet), especially near stairs. If you find one, smooth it out with a runner, a small ramp, or molding.

3. Keep rugs from slipping or curling up at the ends by applying adhesive strips or tacking them down.

4. Put a rubber pad down in front of the kitchen sink where the floor may get wet. In the bathroom, use only rubber-backed mats.

5. Deep pile carpeting can be a hazard for elderly people who use a walker. The front legs of the walker can get caught and cause the person to fall.

Consider installing a textured plastic runner over main passageways, fastened securely.

6. On wooden steps, use adhesive strips or stair treads to prevent slipping.

7. Make sure the outdoor steps are in good repair and their edges are clearly marked or highlighted with strips of colored tape or paint.

8. Make sure outdoor steps have secure railings, and use adhesive strips or flat stair treads to provide a secure surface if steps become slippery when wet.

9. You may wish to install a chair lift (a chair on a rail) for easy, safe movement between floors. Another option is to rearrange the living space so that areas used by the elderly person are all on one floor.

Rug, Carpet, and Stair Checklist

	Basement	First floor	Second floor
Worn or torn rugs?	_____	_____	_____
Changes in walking surface?	_____	_____	_____
Rugs secure?	_____	_____	_____
Rubber mats or backing?	_____	_____	_____
Deep pile carpeting?	_____	_____	_____
Stair treads on wooden steps?	_____	_____	_____
Outdoor steps need repair?	_____	_____	_____
Step edges marked?	_____	_____	_____
Secure railing?	_____	_____	_____
Chair lift needed?	_____	_____	_____

FLOOR SAFETY

1. Make sure wooden or tile surfaces are waxed with a nonskid wax. Also, encourage the elderly to wear slippers with non-skid strips.

2. Clean up wet spots, accidents, or spills as soon as they happen.

3. Keep the floor surface even by flattening out carpet bumps, replacing warped tiles, and fixing any loose or worn stairs.

4. Mark the floor at the top and bottom of steps with reflective tape, and highlight raised thresholds.

5. Get in the habit of immediately picking up toys and other objects that don't belong on the floor. The elderly won't expect them there and may not see them.

6. If needed, construct ramps to ensure safe access to the home or to navigate small level changes in the home.

7. If the home has deep pile carpeting or many transitions between floor levels, consider putting tennis balls over the front feet so that the walker can glide over the carpet. This will minimize the risk of tripping.

Floor Checklist

	Basement	First floor	Second floor
Nonskid wax?	_____	_____	_____
Wet spots?	_____	_____	_____
Smooth surface?	_____	_____	_____
Changes in floor level marked?	_____	_____	_____
Objects in pathway?	_____	_____	_____
Ramps needed?	_____	_____	_____
Special walker needed?	_____	_____	_____

A Family Caregiver's Guide to Planning and Decision Making for the Elderly © 1999 James A. Wilkinson

HANDHOLD AND SUPPORT SAFETY

For the elderly, actions that were once routine—rising from a low chair or toilet seat, or climbing stairs, for example—become difficult and can lead to a fall. This issue is especially important if they tend to lose their balance easily. When people start to fall, their instinct is to grab for support. If nothing is there to grab onto, the person falls awkwardly and may be injured. Strong, well-anchored supports should be placed where the elderly can hold on to them while moving, rising, or shifting positions.

1. There should be handrails on both sides of every stairway. Anchor them to the wall studs about thirty inches from the floor.

2. Stair handrails should extend the entire length of the staircase and, ideally, go beyond the stairs, turning beyond the top or bottom step.

3. Install firmly anchored tub handles to assist climbing in and out of the tub.

4. Install grab bars next to the toilet, especially if it's low or if the person has trouble rising, and anchor them to the wall. Or, install a raised toilet.

5. Chairs should be firm, not soft, and have sturdy arms and legs that can support the person's weight. For chairs without adequate arms, there should be something sturdy close by—not just a table—that the person can hold on to for support while getting into or out of the chair.

Handhold and Support Checklist

	Basement	First floor	Second floor
Handrails secure?	_____	_____	_____
Handrails extend from top of stairs to bottom?	_____	_____	_____
Grab bars next to tub?	_____	_____	_____
Grab bars next to toilet?	_____	_____	_____
Firm, sturdy chairs?	_____	_____	_____
Support nearby for getting in and out of chairs?	_____	_____	_____

FURNITURE AND ACCESSORIES SAFETY

1. Furniture—including beds, sofas, chairs, recliners, and even outdoor furniture—should be comfortable but firm enough that the elderly person doesn't sink into it or have to struggle to get up.

2. Lock the casters or rollers on all furniture. Wheelchairs should have a safety belt and easily accessible brake locks. The locks should always be set, except when the wheelchair is moving.

3. The elderly tend to rock back and forth to create enough momentum to get up, so chairs must be stable enough to support their weight, especially if they use the arms for support when shifting position.

4. Place all items in closets and on shelves within easy reach. Otherwise, place a sturdy step stool with a front or side handrail in the kitchen, pantry, and bath areas so the person can reach shelves easily.

5. If the stairs have a landing that is large enough to hold a chair without blocking the passageway, put a chair there so the elderly person can rest while climbing the stairs.

6. For a frail elderly person, a hospital bed with side rails can provide added security.

7. Pedestal tables, and any other tables that may tip when leaned on, should be moved away from chairs that the elderly use and areas that they walk through.

8. Elderly who live alone should have a telephone next to their bed.

9. Telephones should have large buttons and be easy to use. Adjust the volume so the elderly person can hear the ring as well as the person on the line. Ideally, the home should have at least one cordless phone and an answering machine to screen calls.

10. Near all phones there should be a place to sit down, rest a phone book, and post an emergency contact list. Phone numbers on the emergency contact list should be written large enough to be read without glasses. A pad and pencil should be near the phone to take messages.

11. With the television on, the elderly should still be able to hear the doorbell, the telephone, and someone talking in a normal tone of voice. If they can't, give them some other way to let them know that the doorbell or telephone is ringing (such as a small flashing light).

12. The elderly person's walker should not be so large that he or she has to turn sideways to get through doorways. Also, walkers are not meant for steps. If the person must go up and down steps, there should be a walker on each level.

13. Move electric heaters away from water, curtains, furniture, and anything else that could catch on fire or cause electric shock.

14. For the bedridden elderly, consider using an over-bed table to help them sit up to eat or read.

15. If incontinence is a problem, place a shower curtain or rubber sheet between the sheet and mattress to ease cleanup and protect the mattress.

16. Use foam or sheepskin mats to minimize bed sores or skin tears.

17. Use clocks with large numerals that glow in the dark.

18. Provide reaching devices for things that are too low or too high. Bending and stooping may be as big a problem as reaching up.

A Family Caregiver's Guide to Planning and Decision Making for the Elderly © 1999 James A. Wilkinson

Furniture and Accessories Checklist

	Basement	First floor	Second floor
Can get in and out of furniture?			
Locks on wheels and casters?			
Chairs sturdy and stable?			
Step stool for shelves?			
Chair on landing?			
Hospital bed?			
Pedestal tables out of the way?			
Telephone next to bed?			
Telephones accessible?			
Emergency numbers posted?			
Can hear phone and doorbell?			
Walkers at top and bottom of stairs?			
Electric heater safety?			
Over-bed table?			
Mattress protection?			
Sheepskin to prevent bed sores?			
Glowing clocks?			
Reaching devices?			

DOOR, WINDOW, LOCK, AND ALARM SAFETY

1. On internal doors that are usually closed, consider replacing the knobs with easy-to-use levers.

2. Lock chemicals, cleaners, poisons, and other dangerous items in a safe place. These pose a serious risk for a person with dementia and should be stored in a locked area. Because emergency access to that area may be important, let other people know where the key is hidden.

3. If the elderly person comes and goes from the home, make sure locks are not cumbersome. One good, easy-to-use lock is better than several cheap ones. Check that keys can be turned easily inside locks, that adequate lighting is available, and, if a door has multiple locks, that the elderly person is capable of unlocking and opening the door reasonably quickly.

4. A home security system must be tailored to the elderly person's ability to use it safely. If there's an alarm system, make sure he or she understands how it works, how to turn it off, and what password(s) to use when the security company calls.

5. Smoke and carbon monoxide detectors should be placed near the bedroom and kitchen, at the top of the stairwell, and on each level. If the person doesn't hear well, get an alarm with a flashing light.

6. It may be important for the elderly person to stay in contact with the caregiver, especially if he or she is bedridden or if movement is restricted. Here, an intercom system used to monitor a baby's room can be an inexpensive solution.

7. Lock all windows, but be sure they're not painted shut. In an emergency, the windows should open easily.

8. If the doorways in the house are too narrow for the person's walker or wheelchair, removing some of the doors may give him or her enough room to pass through.

9. Post a copy of the *Personal Safety Precautions* (see page 94).

10. Consider using a personal emergency response system (PERS) or Medic Alert to summon help in an emergency.

Door, Window, Lock, and Alarm Checklist

	Basement	First floor	Second floor
Levers to replace doorknobs?	_____	_____	_____
Dangerous areas locked and keys hidden?	_____	_____	_____
Are keys and locks usable?	_____	_____	_____
Are security system and codes easy to understand?	_____	_____	_____
Smoke detectors?	_____	_____	_____
Intercom needed?	_____	_____	_____
Window locks?	_____	_____	_____
Remove doors?	_____	_____	_____
Safety precautions posted?	_____	_____	_____
PERS or Medic Alert?	_____	_____	_____

KITCHEN SAFETY

In the kitchen, mentally impaired elderly people risk harming themselves and others by the things they might eat, do, or forget to do.

1. In addition to moving items so they're within reach, clearly label all items in the pantry, refrigerator, and freezer.

2. On the stove and oven, the "off" position on the knobs should be clearly marked and easy to see from across the room.

3. Remove any foods the elderly person shouldn't eat. If you simply put them out of reach, you increase the chance that the person will injure himself or herself while trying to reach them. This also applies to other dangerous items, such as alcohol (if the person is taking certain medications) and sharp knives.

4. Furniture should be sturdy, rugs should not slide, and only nonskid wax should be used on the floor.

5. If there's a counter with stools, be sure that the person can get on and off the stools safely. While sitting on a stool, the person's feet should be flat on the ground so he or she can push the stool back from the counter without tilting it.

6. Install temperature locks on faucets to keep the water from getting too hot. You can also lower the water heater temperature.

7. If the elderly person shouldn't use certain appliances, disconnect them or remove them from the home.

8. Keep a small fire extinguisher, with an easy-to-remove pin, within reach.

9. If breakage of china and glassware is a problem, switch to plastic. This will reduce the risk of the elderly cutting themselves.

10. Periodically check the expiration dates on perishable and frozen foods. Circle expiration dates on food packages, and discard any food that is questionable.

11. Many devices are available to help the elderly function safely in the kitchen. Discuss your specific needs with an occupational therapist.

12. Consider buying new appliances with automatic shutoff switches, such as irons or coffee makers.

13. Help the elderly person get in the habit of using a portable timer every time the stove is turned on, even if he or she will be in the kitchen while it's on.

Kitchen Checklist

All items clearly marked and within reach?   _____

"Off" position of stove and oven knobs
visible across the room?   _____

Prohibited items removed?   _____

Rugs secure? Nonskid wax on floor?   _____

Stools safe?   _____

Temperature locks needed?   _____

Prohibited appliances disconnected or removed?   _____

Fire extinguisher handy?   _____

Switch to plastic dishware?   _____

Expiration dates checked on food?   _____

Assistive devices needed?   _____

Appliances with automatic shutoff?   _____

Food timers with loud ring?   _____

BATHROOM SAFETY

1. Install skid-resistant strips and grab bars in the tub, shower, and near the toilet.

2. Unless the unlocked door can be opened with little effort, remove door locks. If a closed door doesn't ensure privacy, get a "Do Not Disturb" sign to hang on the bathroom door when it's in use.

3. Use only rubber-backed or nonskid rugs.

4. Everything in the medicine cabinet should be within reach and clearly labeled. Inappropriate and outdated items should be thrown out.

5. If needed, add a seat to the tub or shower to assist in bathing.

6. Make sure the night light is bright enough to illuminate the room, but not so bright that it causes temporary blindness when the person leaves the room.

7. If standing, reaching, or bending over is a problem, consider a hand-held shower head so the person can sit and bathe.

Bathroom Checklist

Grab bars and skid-resistant strips? _____

Remove door locks? _____

Nonskid rugs? _____

Medicine cabinet safe? _____

Tub or shower seat? _____

Night light? _____

Hand-held shower head? _____

OTHER SAFETY CONCERNS

On this checklist, record any other safety issues, such as the following:

1. Pets. Although pets can offer invaluable companionship, they pose some safety issues, especially when one cat becomes six cats, or when yet another stray dog is adopted. To assess the safety risks, consider the animal's characteristics. Is it large or small? Does it have to go outside, especially at night? Can it go outside alone into an enclosed yard? Does it have accidents in the home? Does it tend to get underfoot? Could it knock the person over? Is it prone to scratch or bite? Can the person manage its care and feeding?

2. Emergency access. In an emergency, could medical workers get to the elderly person and be able to bring him or her out on a stretcher? If the home has narrow halls, tight corners, or steep stairs, critical time can be lost moving the person out of the area or waiting for assistance.

3. Furnace inspection. If the elderly person owns his or her own home or trailer, an annual furnace inspection should be scheduled. (In a condo or apartment complex, the building manager is responsible for the furnace.)

4. Fans. If the elderly person doesn't have air conditioning, make sure there are fans in the home. Check the fans to be sure they provide enough of a breeze to cool the elderly person in warm weather. This is critical in regions that have hot weather for extended periods of time.

Other Safety Concerns Checklist

Pets   _____

Emergency access   _____

Annual furnace inspection   _____

Fans   _____

_____   _____

_____   _____

_____   _____

                                          _____

Personal Safety Precautions

Too often, the news carries stories about elderly people being killed or robbed in their home. Incidents like these may be prevented by taking the following precautions. If the elderly person lives alone, review these safety precautions together and encourage him or her to share them with friends.

These simple safety precautions are for use at home. This is not a comprehensive list. It doesn't cover shopping, driving, or walking safety, for example. However, discussing these issues with the elderly person can get you started on developing your own list of dos and don'ts.

Dos

- Keep outside doors locked at all times.
- Automatically lock windows, car doors, and garage doors.
- Make sure you can see who is at the door without having to open it. If you don't already have a peephole, have one installed.
- Use a telephone answering machine to screen calls. Answer only those calls you want to answer.
- Use timers on lights when you're away. Even when you're home, use them in unused rooms to make it appear that more people are in the house.
- Draw curtains or blinds at night so people can't see in from the outside.
- Invest in a high-quality door lock, ideally a deadbolt that goes into the door frame.
- When you go out, leave a radio, TV, or light on to make it appear that someone is home.
- Set up a check-in system with friends and neighbors. If you go away, let them know how to contact you.
- Keep a copy of your *Vital Information Form* (page 9), an inventory of your possessions (page 26), and all official documents and other important papers in a safety deposit box.
- Update your emergency contact list (pages 215–216) and post it near a telephone for easy access.
- Keep your *Basic Medical Information* (page 57) and *Medication Summary* (page 73) updated, and make copies of each.

Don'ts

- **Don't keep large sums of cash in the home.** If you do, don't let anyone know about it, not even home healthcare and housekeeping workers, family members, friends, or neighbors. If money is missing, report it immediately.

- **Don't let anyone you don't know into your home—** including meter readers, delivery people, or people who want to use the phone in an emergency. If you're expecting a repair person or any other service provider, ask for identification. If someone asks to use your phone because of an emergency, keep the person on the other side of the locked door and make the call yourself. For everyone else, refuse access or ask them to wait until a friend or neighbor can come over. Never let anyone inside when you are alone in the house.

- **Don't indicate that you are away or that you live alone, especially on your answering machine.** Keep the message general: "You have reached 123-4567; please leave a message." Your friends will understand.

- **Don't leave notes on the door or put keys under the mat or in the mailbox when you go out. Likewise, don't let mail and newspapers accumulate at your door.** When you leave town, either stop delivery or arrange for someone to pick them up. If you'll be away for more than a few days, arrange to have the grass cut, the leaves raked, and the snow shoveled to make it look as if someone is home.

- **Don't give money or buy something in response to a "cold call" from a telephone solicitor or stock broker.** Have them send you the information first. Also, discuss gifts and investments with another family member before you make a commitment. Don't be a sucker!

- **Don't fall for lottery or sweepstakes scams.** If you get a phone call from someone who asks you to send in money in order to claim a prize, assume it is a scam and hang up. If you feel threatened, call the police. FBI reports show that more money is stolen over the telephone from the elderly than through armed robbery.

Assessing the Risk of Living at Home

What You Need to Know

The checklists and safety precautions in the last section will help you make an elderly person's home safe and secure. But if there's been a change in his or her physical, mental, or emotional condition, it's possible that no amount of fixing up will be sufficient. A caregiver must look carefully at an elderly person's problems to determine whether independent living is still appropriate or if some level of assistance is needed. In some cases, the elderly may no longer be safe in the home, even with assistance, and new housing may be needed.

If more than one person lives in the home, look at each person's problems and needs individually, and consider what would happen if one person moved out. Let's say, for example, that a married couple lives together in their home. The wife is frail, but quite self-sufficient. Her husband, on the other hand, needs help with basic daily activities, including dressing, bathing, and moving around. Because the wife is no longer able to assist her husband with these activities, their living arrangement is unsafe for both of them. If he were to get intensive home care or move to an assisted-living facility, she could continue living at home. However, if she eventually had to move to a nursing home and he stayed in the house, he would still need constant care and housekeeping services.

Even when one person's condition poses a threat to the other, an elderly couple may not want to be separated after all their years together. However, if either of them is able to understand the issues, you should raise the question of living arrangements. Try to get them to agree that one or both of them has to move. If they insist on staying together and are mentally competent, there is little that you can do, even if one poses a serious risk to the other. However, if one is incompetent, you can ask a court to appoint you his or her legal guardian. If the court agrees, you can then move the elderly person to a safer environment.

What to Look For

Condition of the Home

A home's physical condition may be the first sign of potential problems. Signs of neglect may indicate that a clean and safe home is more than the person can handle, either physically or financially. If it's just a matter of upkeep (such as uncut grass and dirty windows) or minor maintenance (such as peeling paint), there may be no need to worry. It could mean that the home's appearance is simply no longer important to the elderly person. However, if there's structural damage to the home, it's time to be concerned.

Piles of dirty dishes; the odor of urine or excrement (whether human or animal); an infestation of bugs or roaches; evidence of rodents or animal damage; a filthy bathroom; spoiled food in the refrigerator or pantry; dirty clothes, sheets, and towels; broken appliances or fixtures—all are strong evidence that the person is no longer capable of living alone safely. Whether the danger is physical (as in the risk of fire or falling) or involves quality of life (inadequate nutrition, lack of heat), you should consider alternative housing or, at the least, intensive home care or housekeeping services.

Behavior

In some cases, the home may be fine, but the elderly may show signs of inappropriate thinking or behavior—having no food in the house, turning the furnace off in the winter, storing the iron in the refrigerator, acquiring unnecessary items (two refrigerators, four televisions, and a new set of encyclopedias, for example), and so on. Other times, the elderly person's behavior doesn't change, but friends sense there's a problem, even if they can't articulate what it is. When an elderly person's behavior or personality changes, he or she will likely be unaware of its significance, and others may dismiss it as an eccentricity. The fact is, changes like these are serious and should be monitored.

In addition to the obvious, look for more subtle signs that assistance may be needed. Check the pantry and refrigerator to see if the elderly person is eating three meals a day. Malnutrition is a common problem among the elderly, especially as their ability to perform routine activities deteriorates. Do you see any unpaid bills or utility shut-off notices? Is the elderly person getting calls from bill collectors? Are objects disappearing from the home? Do you find that there's not enough money to pay the bills, even though there should be?

Do you find packages containing worthless gifts or prizes? Have there been any calls from people who will only speak with the elderly person, or who tell you that more prizes have been won? These are signs that the person is being victimized by a scam or fraud.

Because the elderly are often victims of "contractor" fraud, you might also be concerned if the person becomes involved in a major home-remodeling project. Sometimes the services are paid for but never provided. In other cases, a small problem turns into a major repair. Tell the elderly person that you would like to discuss any remodeling projects before he or she signs a contract or makes a nonrefundable deposit. If you suspect the person is being victimized, don't hesitate to contact the local postal inspector or police, even if a contract has been signed and the work has already been done.

Physical, mental, and emotional problems are also signs that some level of assistance is needed. Any of the following behaviors should cause immediate concern. The elderly:

• Can't remember if or how much medication they took, or they forget to take their medication altogether.

• Are unkempt, dirty, or smelly, or they refuse to dress appropriately, change clothes, or bathe.

• Report falling, or show evidence of a fall, but minimize the problem or can't remember it happening.

• Fail to eat regularly or properly, for any reason. Be concerned if they can't remember how to cook, when to eat, if they have eaten, or what they ate. Any sudden weight loss or evidence of malnutrition or dehydration may indicate a serious problem.

• Appear to be lip reading; fail to acknowledge the telephone, the doorbell, or a knock at the door; or don't respond to a sudden, loud noise. An undiagnosed hearing deficit is a serious safety problem.

• Have problems with any of the Activities of Daily Living or Intermediate Activities of Daily Living (see page 76).

• Show fear of living alone or of another person. Fear should be dealt with immediately, especially when accompanied by mysterious lumps, bruises, or skin tears.

• Tend to wander out of the home or dress inappropriately for the weather.

• Become reclusive and spend hours in a bedroom or darkened room.

• Don't make sense when answering simple questions.

• Insist on driving even when it poses a risk to themselves and others.

• Appear to be abusing alcohol or medications, including over-the-counter medications.

• Smoke in the house, despite a tendency to nod off or fall asleep while smoking.

• Suddenly begin adopting stray pets and insist that it's okay to live with more than two dogs or cats.

• Show a major personality change, especially violent outbursts, striking others, verbal abuse, or swearing.

• Forget recent phone calls or visitors.

Social Contacts

How isolated is the elderly person? Do you know who his or her friends are and how to contact them? Is the person an active part of the community? Does he or she get calls or visits from friends, neighbors, caregivers, or clergy? How often does the elderly person get out of the home to shop, go to church, or visit friends? Is the community relatively safe, or is the person locked in the home and afraid of going out, even during the day? If he or she remains at home, will home care and housekeeping services be easy to arrange? If the person has become reclusive and has little contact with people outside the home, continuing to live alone could be dangerous.

A Geriatric Assessment

It is difficult to be objective when assessing the physical, mental, and emotional health of a person you care for. Caregivers may be overly sensitive to minor problems, while minimizing severe impairments to avoid facing the fact that the elderly person's condition is declining. Even if a caregiver tries to be objective, it's hard to know how to measure an elderly person's condition. For these reasons, a comprehensive geriatric assessment may be needed at some point.

If the purpose for the assessment is to determine whether or not the elderly person can continue living at home, request a home visit. Most urban and community hospitals have teams of doctors, nurses,

therapists, nutritionists, and social workers who specialize in geriatric care and can perform assessments in the home. They can determine if it's safe to continue living independently, if in-home assistance is needed, or if a more appropriate living arrangement is necessary.

Involving the Family

Try to get everyone to agree up front that an independent assessment is needed, and to abide by the outcome. If another caregiver or family member strongly opposes the idea of an independent assessment, it can lead to state involvement, litigation, and perhaps a family feud. If there is opposition at the start, don't assume that everyone will suddenly become rational and agree to "do the right thing" just because they've read the assessor's report.

If the elderly person is mentally competent but absolutely refuses to cooperate, you must proceed cautiously. Encourage him or her to talk to a physician. A physician may be able to convince the person to reconsider his or her decision. If the elderly person still refuses to participate, there is little you can do.

Keep in mind that the more evidence you collect to verify specific problems with the elderly person and his or her living conditions, the easier it will be for others—including the elderly—to accept the conclusions of the assessment. Ultimately, the facts are what they are. The best way to reach a consensus is to help everyone involved confront those facts. Remember, unless it's an emergency, a geriatric assessment will take time. This time can be used to forge consensus within the family.

Assessment Results

If the geriatric assessment doesn't turn up any major problems, and the living environment is basically okay, there's no reason to upset the status quo if the elderly person doesn't want to move or doesn't want in-home assistance. Although you may want to investigate housing options for the future, don't force a change when one isn't clearly warranted.

However, if the geriatric assessment reveals problems that can't be corrected with in-home assistance, it's time to select a more appropriate living arrangement (see chapter 5). You'll need to decide where the elderly person will live and how much time you have to make the change. In general, the sooner the move is made, the better.

The assessment may show that the elderly person can continue to live at home, but only with assistance. If this is the case, there are a number of eldercare services and assistive devices designed to help the elderly live safely and comfortably in their home. The following section explains how to assist an elderly person who lives at home, and how to get the caregiving help you need.

Assisting an Elderly Person Who Lives at Home

What You Need to Know

Keeping the elderly safe in their home may involve a variety of family, professional, and community resources. Those resources may range from routine maintenance, such as mowing the lawn, to the use of assistive devices or sophisticated medical services.

If you decide that the elderly person can continue to live safely at home, but only with help, you will need to help him or her define the level and type of assistance needed. This section will give you details about assistive devices and the role of volunteer and professional caregivers. Later you will read about the range of services and benefits available in most communities, as well as the process for selecting home healthcare, home care, and housekeeping service providers.

Assistive Devices

As people age, their balance and strength may be affected as well as their ability to bend over, reach up, see, hear, speak, and move around. Assistive devices are tools and other instruments that help people compensate for their limitations and perform routine tasks safely and comfortably. Many elderly people who live alone require some assistive devices to meet everyday needs around the house.

Once a problem has been identified, social workers, therapists, hospital discharge planners, contractors, home service centers, consumer magazines, and catalogs can suggest devices that might help. You will need to know where to buy them, how much they cost, and if a third party will help pay for them. Devices may be simple and inexpensive, such as jar openers or dishes with suction cups on the bottom to prevent sliding, or they can be costly, like a portable oxygen system or a custom-designed chair lift for going up and down stairs. Assistive devices can be found in hardware stores, discount chains, drug stores, home service centers, and medical supply companies. If necessary, they should be installed by a professional.

When considering assistive devices, keep in mind the following:

1. Before you buy anything, examine the problem you're trying to solve. Assistive devices tend to be more helpful with physical problems than mental problems. Therefore, it's essential to understand the underlying issues. For example, if the elderly person won't get into the tub for fear of falling, grab bars may help. But if the underlying problem is dementia, and the person doesn't understand the need for a bath, grab bars won't help.

2. Make sure the device will alleviate the problem. Before purchasing an assistive device, try it out yourself. Then make sure that the elderly person can and will use it. If it's too complicated, too heavy, or too awkward, he or she probably won't use it again. This is especially true for electronic items and appliances. For someone with dementia, even a simple device like a television remote control can be too difficult to use.

3. Try to meet the elderly person's preferences as well as his or her needs. If the elderly person wants a device that is sturdy, easy to clean, light enough to carry, and green to match the room, try to find a device that meets all these criteria. Also, make sure that the device will fit where it needs to go. You don't want to sacrifice safety, but if you sacrifice seemingly nonessential attributes, you may find that the person will refuse to use the device.

4. Make sure the device won't make the problem worse. For example, if an elderly person has significant problems with balance or strength, installing grab bars next to the tub may simply increase the chance of a fall. This person doesn't need a device; he or she needs personal assistance. Don't install an assistive device that might encourage an elderly person to try to do something he or she can't do safely.

5. Make sure the device is properly installed, and don't throw away the items you replace. If installation is required, make sure it's done by a qualified person or contractor according to the manufacturer's specifications and local building codes. If the assistive device is installed improperly, the elderly person could be severely hurt if it fails. Also, keep the old fixtures so they can be reinstalled if you sell the home.

6. Save the packing box and receipt so you can return the device if it doesn't work or isn't used. You may have to go through a process of trial and error to find out what devices will work and what the elderly person can and will use. The store may not take a device back, but try to return it anyway, especially if it was never used.

7. Find out if a third party will help pay for the device. If a device is medically necessary and prescribed by a doctor, it may be covered by Medicare, Medicaid, or insurance. Generally, the medical equipment or supply company can tell you if you're likely to be reimbursed. The less medical the item, the less likely it is to be covered. If you're installing the device as part of a large home improvement project, a federal or community home improvement program may help fund it. Either way, it's best to treat every purchase as an out-of-pocket expense so you're not inconvenienced if a third-party refuses to pay for it.

8. Consult a therapist from your local rehabilitation clinic. If the elderly person develops a physical problem and you aren't sure what to do, contact your local rehabilitation clinic or hospital. Even if the elderly person isn't a patient there, you can often pay a rehabilitation therapist to make a home visit. He or she will do a home assessment and may be able to recommend useful assistive devices.

Volunteer Caregivers

While assistive devices play a crucial role in keeping the elderly at home, their role is limited. Most in-home care to frail elderly people is supplied by volunteer caregivers. A volunteer caregiver is usually a female family member who lives with or near the elderly person. The caregiver ensures that the elderly person's needs are met, coordinates in-home services, acts as the primary contact person for service providers and the family, and balances the elderly person's needs with the resources available to meet them.

One of the most important issues caregivers face is balance—weighing what they can do for the elderly person against what others can do. They must decide which home care and housekeeping services to do themselves, and which to contract to outside providers. The decision depends on the elderly person's needs, the caregiver's time and ability, how much money is available to pay for assistance, and what types of services can be provided in the elderly person's home or within the community. Relying on outside services can create stress and may be misunderstood by others, but if the caregiving relationship is going to be long term, it's essential to get other people involved.

Personally providing daily care can be stressful, putting the caregiver's mental and physical health at risk. Although this problem often goes unrecognized, the caregiver's health and well-being is as important as the elderly person's. Literature on caregiving is full of warnings not to try to do it all. Caregivers must have regular relief from their responsibilities. They must also learn to focus on what is important and turn the rest over to other people. If there isn't enough money to hire care services, assistance from family and friends is a must. If that help is unavailable, other housing alternatives should be pursued immediately.

Hiring a Professional

If you can afford it, you might consider hiring a geriatric care manager or social worker who specializes in home care (see chapter 7). Professional care managers can assist the primary caregiver or coordinate caregiving services. However, they generally charge by the hour, and their fees must fit into the caregiving budget.

Geriatric care managers have two advantages: a detailed knowledge of community resources and a personal relationship with those resources. This is important, because few communities have an informative, one-stop helpline or referral source for home healthcare, home care, and housekeeping services. Finding help on your own is often a difficult, time-consuming process. If you don't know what services you need or what questions to ask,

you could make the process more difficult—and you may end up hiring the wrong provider. This is where a geriatric care manager can help. He or she can translate the elderly person's needs into a coordinated plan of support. Furthermore, a geriatric care manager may inspire service providers to do a better job, since providers want to impress care managers in order to get future referrals.

If you hire a professional, make sure your expectations are realistic. Remember, even the experts will take vacations, get sick, and have other problems. They might also have responsibilities to other clients.

Whether or not you hire a professional, it's wise to explore other services available for the elderly. A number of these are discussed in the pages that follow.

Services Available for the Elderly

The following is a list of services available in most communities, although their labels may vary. For more on selecting a service provider, refer to Selecting In-Home Care Providers on page 111.

Adult daycare

Adult daycare is an option for elderly people living at home who need therapeutic support or rehabilitative services in a structured setting several days a week. Services may include nursing, personal care, health assessment, vaccinations, social services, meals, rehabilitation, and transportation. Special programs may be offered for those with dementia or Alzheimer's disease. The noon meal is often included in the daily charge. Although these programs are structured to assist the elderly, they also provide a needed break for the primary caregiver.

Carrier alert

At most post offices, an elderly person can register an emergency number for mail carriers to call if they notice mail accumulating in the person's mailbox.

Companionship

Companions, or friendly visitors, visit elderly people who live alone and are isolated or homebound. They can provide conversation and assistance with light errands or housekeeping. Sometimes escort services are included, where companions transport and accompany the elderly on errands or doctor visits. Companions aren't trained for medical or personal care and do not typically perform housekeeping duties.

Congregate care meals

These programs offer the elderly a nutritious meal at a school, senior center, or community facility. The elderly must have their own transportation, and a contribution or minimal payment may be required. Meals are often combined with free recreational or educational programs.

Emergency response

These services provide twenty-four-hour emergency help for individuals who are at high risk for falling, accidents, or other medical emergencies. Usually, button-activated devices are used to send a help signal to a central response center, which alerts emergency personnel. These services also include medical identification tags or cards.

Handyman

These services include light and heavy housekeeping, minor repairs, yard work, snow removal, leaf cleanup, window washing, home winterization, assistive device installation, and many other tasks.

Home care

Home care, or homemaker, services include laundry, shopping, light cleaning, meal preparation, personal assistance and care, escorting, and other nonhealth-related services. Any of these can offer tremendous relief to the primary caregiver. Home care is discussed in greater detail on page 107.

Home healthcare

Home healthcare services include any kind of in-home nursing, social work, or rehabilitation therapy, including physical, occupational, respiratory, or recreational therapy. These services can be provided by an agency or an independent provider. Home healthcare services are discussed in greater detail on page 104.

Hospital supply

Hospital supply companies, durable medical equipment suppliers, and home healthcare companies will sell or lease assistive devices, medical supplies, and other equipment, including canes, walkers, oxygen systems, hospital beds, ostomy supplies, and bath chairs.

Housekeeping

Housekeeping services are essentially the same as home care services, except no personal care is involved. Some handyman services may also be offered, however. Housekeeping services are discussed in greater detail on page 107.

Housing assistance

These services help the elderly find senior congregate care, shared housing, or emergency shelter. They may be sponsored by a nonprofit organization or by a government office, such as your local housing authority or Area Agency on Aging.

Meals-on-Wheels

This is a generic term for any home-delivered meal program. These programs offer nutritional hot or cold meals to the homebound elderly once or twice a day. Some of these programs are free or heavily subsidized by a local church or government; others require payment based on a sliding scale.

PAL

Some communities have a phone assistance league (PAL), which elderly people check in with each day. If PAL doesn't receive this daily call, a volunteer will try to contact the elderly person and summon emergency personnel to the person's home if there's no answer.

Senior centers

These centers offer recreational, educational, and social services to the mobile elderly. A few services, such as transportation or meals, may be provided free of charge. These centers are also an excellent source of information about local resources for the elderly, including health screening.

Social daycare

Social daycare offers recreational, social, and support services in a structured setting five days a week. These services typically do not include rehabilitation or therapy, but may offer transportation and health monitoring.

Telephone reassurance

These services offer phone calls daily—or more often, if necessary—by volunteers who provide reassurance and socialization to the isolated or homebound elderly. Volunteers may also keep a chart on medication usage, nutritional information, or medical appointments. As with carrier alert and PAL services, if an elderly person fails to answer the phone, a volunteer will go to his or her home or send an emergency response team.

Transportation

A number of public and private organizations offer free or discounted transportation to a variety of destinations, especially those related to health or congregate care.

In addition to these, the elderly may be entitled to other services mentioned in this book, including Social Security, Supplemental Security Income (SSI), veterans benefits, pensions, and general entitlement benefits such as food stamps and discounted services. For programs that can assist with home repairs, see chapter 7 or contact Christmas in April (page 228). For information on subsidized housing, read page 123.

Check with your state Area Agency on Aging (page 241) to see what other free or discounted programs are available in your state or community. Ask about adult education, discount medication programs, driver's license discounts, protection from abuse, tax assistance or relief, transportation, and utility bill rebates or discounts. And, don't forget the senior citizen discounts offered by many merchants.

While many eldercare services take place in a variety of settings, the most common services—home healthcare, home care, and housekeeping services—take place in the elderly person's home. The remainder of this chapter is devoted to these types of in-home services.

Planning Home Healthcare

What You Need to Know

The home healthcare business is often difficult for the consumer to sort out because there are no established standards or certifying authorities. While there are many reputable providers, fraud is not uncommon. The best way to begin your search is with a firm recommendation from a reputable source. The Yellow Pages may be a good place to find tires, but it isn't the best place to find a home healthcare provider.

If the elderly person is being discharged from the hospital, a hospital discharge planner may be your best source of information. You also can get referrals from geriatric care managers, the elderly person's doctor, your local Area Agency on Aging, the elderly person's insurer, social service agencies, friends, public health services, and your local Visiting Nurses Association.

If you're working with a hospital discharge planner or geriatric care manager, he or she will identify qualified providers for you. If you're looking for a provider on your own, however, you may have to make a decision quickly, and with little information. Therefore, it pays to be organized, keep good notes, focus on one or two leading candidates, and know what questions to ask. (See Selecting In-Home Care Providers on page 111.)

Short-Term vs. Long-Term Care

Duration of assistance is a critical issue. If the elderly person is recovering from hip replacement surgery, he or she may need home healthcare and home care services for only a month or two. However, if the elderly person has had a stroke and is permanently immobilized, you will face a completely different set of issues. The longer the service is required, the more it will cost. Also, if the problem is long-term, the service will need to be monitored, often on a daily basis, which creates more stress on the caregiver.

It is important to determine the level of progress you expect to see. Before selecting home healthcare services, talk to the elderly person's doctor. Can you expect the elderly person to be walking on his or her own within three months? Can you expect the elderly person to be able to go up and down stairs safely?

Cost

Although the goal is to keep the elderly person living at home, you have to compare the cost of home healthcare with the cost of other options, including alternative housing. Try to fully estimate the cost of each alternative before you make a firm commitment to one or the other.

Home Healthcare Providers

The medical needs of the homebound elderly are usually met through either a home healthcare agency or individual healthcare professionals. Typically, in-home services are provided by nurses, therapists, or home healthcare aides.

• **Registered nurses (RNs)** are highly trained professionals who can provide a wide range of services. Because they are expensive and few cases require their level of skill, RNs aren't usually involved in daily caregiving. RNs are generally involved in assessing elderly needs, developing care plans, or overseeing the services provided by others. In a small community, however, an RN may provide caregiving during the day while a home healthcare aide takes over in the evening.

• **Licensed practical nurses (LPNs) and licensed vocational nurses (LVNs)** are nurses with several years of training. They can provide nursing care under the direction of a registered nurse or a doctor.

- **Home healthcare aides** provide the majority of routine home healthcare to the elderly. This may involve feeding, dressing, bathing, and changing bandages as well as nonmedical chores such as light housework or shopping. Specially trained aides can assist with exercise and skin care, including the treatment of bed sores.

- **Companions** have virtually no healthcare training, but they are able to provide companionship as well as help with meal preparation and housekeeping. To reduce the cost of twenty-four-hour care, some people use companions for the night shift (with a doctor's permission) to provide routine assistance and summon help if necessary.

- **Therapists** provide a range of services, depending on their specialty. Actual in-home services are usually performed by assistants or technicians, who have less training and are less expensive, but therapists are often involved in developing the care plan.

- **Physical therapists** seek to restore movement and bodily control with the use of assistive devices and exercises that improve strength, muscle tone, flexibility, and balance.

- **Occupational therapists** help the elderly compensate for physical limitations, whether caused by a chronic condition (such as arthritis) or a sudden event (like a stroke). They use exercises and other activities to improve mental and physical strength, dexterity, and independence.

- **Speech therapists** seek to improve language or speech skills that have been impaired by illness, disease, or injury. They use assistive devices that enhance the person's ability to understand and communicate, as well as exercises to improve his or her physical abilities.

- **Respiratory therapists** use breathing equipment, such as ventilators and portable oxygen systems, and teach techniques and exercises to maintain proper respiration.

Agencies vs. Individual Providers

Home healthcare providers can generally be divided into two categories: agencies and individuals. Each has advantages and disadvantages:

AGENCIES

Advantages

- One agency usually can provide all the medical and personal care services you may need
- A contract that explains services and costs
- One weekly or monthly payment
- Agency handles Social Security and income tax withholding, workers' compensation, insurance, bonding, and other personnel issues
- Temporary personnel available to fill in when others are sick or on vacation
- If Medicare-certified, may provide some personal care in addition to skilled nursing services

Disadvantages

- Personnel are shifted as agency priorities and workloads change, often without notice
- The employee's primary relationship is with the agency, not the elderly person
- Varying degrees of skill and diverse backgrounds among employees
- Little or no choice in which worker will provide the care

INDIVIDUALS

Advantages

- Closer relationship between caregiver and elderly person

- Familiarity with the worker you hire
- Usually lower cost, because there's no administrative overhead

Disadvantages
- Potential problems with sick days, weekends, and vacations of care worker
- Narrow specialty, so the worker may not be able to identify a need for other services
- More payments, especially if several workers are involved
- Employer must handle income tax and Social Security withholding, employee benefits, workers' compensation, and bonding issues
- Lack of accreditation for Medicare
- Problems with turnover, competence, dependability, and compatibility between the worker and elderly person must be handled by the caregiver

Arranging Care after a Hospital Stay

In-home medical services may be required at any time; however, they are most often needed after a hospital stay. When a person is admitted to the hospital, both Medicare and managed care organizations will pay only for a certain number of days. As the payment period comes to an end, the hospital discharge planner must find a way to meet the patient's continuing medical needs. This will often involve home healthcare.

Before the patient is discharged from the hospital, if the expected need for care or therapy is extensive, you should explore some of the residential housing options discussed in chapter 5. All of these services should be available in your community, although they may be listed under different names. You should also explore the possibility of continued insurance coverage, such as Medicare's skilled nursing coverage.

Don't allow the patient to leave the hospital until you have a plan in place to meet his or her medical needs. A person who needs ongoing medical care should never go home until the in-home medical care providers have been hired. To arrange this home care, use the hospital's social work or discharge planning office for recommendations.

For example, even if the elderly person has had outpatient surgery, he or she may be discharged in a medically unstable condition. Make sure that support is available in case an unexpected complication develops after the patient returns home. Having a home healthcare aide on hand for the first twenty-four hours could prevent an ambulance trip back to the hospital—as well as the ensuing insurance hassle.

If you don't know whether medical assistance will be needed, hire the service anyway. Be sure you can cancel it if it isn't needed. Better to arrange it beforehand than try to find a provider with no time to compare services, check references, interview providers, or negotiate prices.

Ask the doctor what in-home medical care the patient will need after he or she leaves the hospital. Then, find out if Medicare, Medicaid, or insurance will help cover the cost. Remember, a third party may be more likely to pay for products or services that have been "ordered" by a doctor. If in doubt, consult an expert at the doctor's office, hospital, or home healthcare agency. If the service you need is covered by Medicare, you would not only save money, but also limit your search for home healthcare to Medicare-certified providers. If there is any chance that a service or product may qualify for third-party payment, be sure to satisfy all approval and prenotification requirements before the patient leaves the hospital.

Monitoring Home Healthcare

As the primary caregiver, you need to continually assess all aspects of the elderly person's condition to see if his or her needs have changed. This means reviewing the person's physical, mental, emotional, and financial condition, as well as his or her living environment. It also means monitoring in-home services to be sure that needs and expectations are being met. Schedule regular doctor visits and periodically review the *Medication List* (page 70) and Activities of Daily Living (pages 76–78). Remember that any change in the ADLs should be discussed with a doctor.

As the elderly person's needs change, the need for home healthcare may also change. Continually review the need for in-home services, especially if they're covered by a third party. Third-party payments will almost always end after a certain period of time, and you'll need to have a backup plan in case the services are still needed. Periodically ask yourself the following questions:

- What will happen when this service ends?
- For how much longer might this service be needed?
- How would the service be paid for?
- What are our other options?

The more the elderly person needs a service, the more important it is to confront these issues before third-party payments end, and the more urgent it is to consider other options, such as alternative financing or a new living arrangement. It is difficult—if not impossible—to raise funds overnight or to find immediate placement in a desirable living facility. With the case of moving the elderly person to an assisted-living facility, for example, there may be waiting lists and admission requirements that will delay the move.

Planning Home Care and Housekeeping Services

What You Need to Know

Although some elderly people never need home healthcare, almost all will need home care and housekeeping services at some point. If the elderly person's finances, home environment, or physical or mental condition deteriorate, chances are good that he or she will need help with household chores.

Many caregivers will provide these services themselves; however, hiring professionals to take over some of these responsibilities will give caregivers a much-needed break. Home care services may include yard work, snow removal, home maintenance, housekeeping, window cleaning, cooking, shopping, transportation, laundry, pet care, and bill paying.

Hiring home care and housekeeping services is slightly different from hiring home healthcare services. With home healthcare, licensed professionals are paid to meet clearly identified medical needs for a defined period of time, and the service may be paid for by insurance or governmental support. Home care and housekeeping services, however, are more open-ended arrangements, especially regarding the duration that services are performed. And, with the exception of services provided by volunteers or nonprofit organizations, home care and housekeeping services are almost always paid for by the elderly person or caregiver.

You might hire home care and housekeeping services yourself (see Selecting In-Home Providers beginning on page 111), or you can rely on a geriatric care manager to organize the services for you. (Geriatric care managers generally won't perform the services personally; they will hire other providers.) In either case, you must know who is responsible for the service and hold them accountable for the results. (Also see Finding Local Resources on page 115.)

How to Use the *Home Care and Housekeeping Form*

Home care and housekeeping services must be monitored closely. When several services are provided at once, however, this can be a challenge. To ensure that all the elderly person's needs are being met, use the *Home Care and Housekeeping Form*. If you keep it updated, this form will serve as a handy reference when you need to replace a service provider or find a backup worker when someone calls in sick.

On the first line in each section, describe one of the elderly person's needs in detail. Start with those needs identified in the *Activities of Daily Living Checklist* (page 77), such as "needs help with shoes and buttons" or "can't prepare meals" and go from there. Then, think about the elderly person's home care and housekeeping needs. List each need separately, and be as comprehensive as possible. This could be a long list.

On the second line, indicate if the need could be met outside the elderly person's home. Some meals, for example, could be provided at your local senior center. Many community services can meet a person's needs while providing an opportunity to socialize, which can be equally important.

On the third line, indicate how the need is currently being met and whether or not that solution is adequate. For example, the elderly person may still cook, but if he or she heats up frozen macaroni and cheese for dinner every night, a Meals-on-Wheels program may provide more nutritious meals.

On the fourth line, indicate providers you have hired and any community organizations, services, or agencies that could help you meet that need. It's generally a good idea to rely on as few providers as possible. The fewer people you have to interview, hire, and monitor, the better. It can be difficult and stressful to constantly arrange for substitutes or replacements.

On the fifth line, record telephone numbers, names, backup options, and any other comments that will make this form useful to you.

HOME CARE AND HOUSEKEEPING FORM

Need _____

Home or community? _____

How need is being met _____

Providers _____

Comments _____

Need _____

Home or community? _____

How need is being met _____

Providers _____

Comments _____

Need _____

Home or community? _____

How need is being met _____

Providers _____

Comments _____

Need _____

Home or community? _____

How need is being met _____

Providers _____

Comments _____

Need _____

Home or community? _____

How need is being met _____

Providers _____

Comments _____

Need_____

Home or community? _____

How need is being met _____

Providers _____

Comments _____

Need_____

Home or community? _____

How need is being met _____

Providers _____

Comments _____

Need_____

Home or community? _____

How need is being met _____

Providers _____

Comments _____

Need_____

Home or community? _____

How need is being met _____

Providers _____

Comments _____

Need_____

Home or community? _____

How need is being met _____

Providers _____

Comments _____

Selecting In-Home Care Providers

What You Need to Know

Eventually, most caregivers will need to hire in-home service providers. These providers will come into the elderly person's home and, in some cases, become involved in the most personal aspects of his or her life. Therefore, providers must be carefully screened and monitored. You want the elderly to receive the best possible care, which means you'll have to hire the best possible providers. (If you are a long-distance caregiver, also refer to Caregiving from a Distance on page 115.)

Whenever possible, include the elderly person in the hiring decision. This will eliminate any uncertainty or confusion in his or her mind about why a professional caregiver is needed. It will also help clarify everyone's expectations. The success of in-home services depends, in part, on the elderly person accepting that the provider is a paid professional, not a slave. Otherwise, he or she may refuse to accept the provider or make unreasonable or inappropriate demands, impairing the provider's ability to do his or her job.

Before You Begin ...

The first step in selecting a service provider is to gather information. It's usually best to do this over the telephone. To make the process easier and more efficient, use the following guidelines:

1. Get organized. If you are hiring for home healthcare, talk to the elderly person's doctor about what kind of care is needed and for how long. Otherwise, fill out the *Home Care and Housekeeping Form* on page 109 to clarify and prioritize the issues you need to address. Next, make a list of prospective providers and their phone numbers. Finally, write down a list of questions to ask each provider (see page 112 for ideas). Keep a separate pad of paper nearby to record the answers.

2. Call first thing in the morning. By calling early in the day, you have the opportunity to share any information you get with the doctor, the elderly person, and other family members that same day. You also stand a better chance of reaching the person you need to talk to. If you get a voicemail recording, don't leave a message unless you have to. Speak to an operator if you have that option, and ask to stay on hold until the person you're calling is available.

3. State your questions or request clearly—for example, to get information, schedule a meeting, or speak to a particular person. If the person you're speaking to can't help you, ask if he or she can refer you to someone else. Never pass up an opportunity to network.

4. Keep your questions and answers short. Remember, these people have other things to do. If they're in business or sales, they won't need to know the elderly person's medical history. Just ask them about their services. Answer their questions, but don't get bogged down. Keep the conversation moving.

5. Don't waste time trying to take down every detail. Make general notes and expand on them after you hang up. Use a separate sheet of paper to record each call, so you don't confuse your notes later.

6. If potential providers say anything that excludes them from further consideration, end the call politely. For example, if you know Medicare will pay for the service you're seeking, and you find out that the agency you're talking to isn't Medicare-certified, there's no reason to ask any more questions. However, always keep your contact notes, in case you need to talk to the provider later about another kind of service.

7. Never make a commitment based on a conversation with a salesperson. Review the details of important documents, such as fee schedules and contracts, and talk to an elderlaw attorney before you commit to anything. Ask to have information mailed or faxed to you. If it will take too long to have the information mailed, be prepared to give out a fax number. If you don't have a fax machine, get permission to use a friend's fax machine and give out that number, or give the number of a fax service.

8. Be polite but forceful in seeking answers and clarifying information. Don't end a call until you have the information you need.

Questions for Providers

You may want to ask the following questions when you talk to providers. Some of these questions may not be relevant to your situation, so you may prefer to make up your own list.

When speaking to home healthcare providers, you will need to have the elderly person's Social Security number, his or her Medicare claim number, any supplemental health insurance information, the doctor's orders, and the care plan, if one exists. (A care plan is developed by a hospital discharge planner before the elderly person leaves the hospital. It sets forth the kind of care that will be needed after the person is discharged.) Based on your discussions with the elderly person's doctor, you should also know exactly what services you need, and for approximately how long. For example, "skilled nursing services during the day, including weekends, for three weeks."

Home Healthcare Providers

• "How long have you been in the home healthcare business?" (For agencies: "Do you operate statewide, regionally, or nationally?") This may be an indication of financial strength and quality.

• "Are you state-licensed to provide this service?"

• "Are you Medicare-certified? Are you a Medicaid provider? Are you an approved provider for (the elderly person's health insurance carrier)?"

• "Are you accredited? By whom? Since when?" Accreditation by the National Association of Home Care is a mark of quality.

• "Do you provide (skilled nursing care, respiratory services, home care, and so on)?" Be specific about your needs. If you are unsure of the elderly person's medical needs, speak with his or her doctor first.

• "Is there a written description of each service, what it includes, and its cost? Are additional services billed separately?" Here you are trying to find out if there are any hidden fees or charges. If the service is covered in full by Medicare or insurance, you don't need to ask this question.

• "If Medicare payment is denied, do you handle the appeal? Will we have to pay the charge while the appeal is pending?"

• "How often will the elderly person be billed? Are all charges and the dates of service shown on the invoice? What are the payment terms?"

• "Are any of the charges tax-deductible?"

• "Do we have any control over the selection of the in-home worker?"

• "Will we have the same care worker each time, or do care workers rotate? Can we change care workers if we want to?"

• "Will a formal care plan be given to the doctor and primary care worker in order to manage and evaluate the services?"

• "Will we be involved in developing and implementing the care plan?"

• "Who will explain the care plan to the family?"

• "How do you measure the quality of care provided? How do you measure the elderly person's progress?"

• "Who conducts initial and follow-up assessments of the elderly person? How often is an in-home assessment done?"

Home Care and Housekeeping Services

- "How long have you been in business?"
- "How do you select, train, and monitor the performance of your employees?"
- "What services do you arrange or provide (home healthcare, personal care, home care, housekeeping, and so on)?"
- "Can we interview the employees who will be providing care?"
- "Can we change care workers if we want to?"
- "Are your fees negotiable?"

All Providers

- "Do you put your estimates and fees in writing?"
- "Will you send us a copy of your contract?"
- "How can we end the contractual arrangement?"
- "Are all your employees bonded and covered by your workers' compensation and malpractice insurance?" When you hire an independent contractor from an agency, you may be liable if he or she is injured in the home or has items stolen from the home. If you are unsure about the risks involved in hiring a healthcare provider, seek help from an elderlaw attorney.
- "Do you have a document that sets forth the rights and responsibilities of the patient, the care worker, and the agency?"
- "Whom do we contact with complaints, problems, and requests?"
- "Whom do we contact if the care worker doesn't show up or if there's an emergency?"
- "How do you handle vacations, holidays, and sick days?"
- Ask for three references whom you may contact, including at least one that is no more than a month old.
- If the agency has provided services to someone with a similar problem, ask if you can contact that person or his or her family. To protect patient confidentiality, the agency may refuse or need time to get permission before giving out the name.

How to Choose a Provider
Checking References

Once you have narrowed your options down to one or two choices, check each candidate's references. For an agency, check with the Better Business Bureau or its local equivalent, your referral sources, and other families who have hired the agency. For individual providers, get the person's full name, a copy of his or her Social Security card, his or her address and phone number, and the names of several references. Check as many personal and professional references as you can. If the provider will work unsupervised, also check if he or she has a criminal record. The less you know about the person, the more references you should get.

Interviews

After you've checked references, select one or two service providers for personal interviews. Try to schedule these interviews with the people who would provide the actual service. This may not be possible with an agency, since you could have a different healthcare provider each week. But if you're hiring an individual, a personal interview is a must. Try to involve the elderly person in each interview, if possible.

Call to confirm the interview ahead of time. This will impress the importance of the interview on the other person. Get your notes in order and determine if you have any particular questions or issues to discuss.

During the interview, describe your needs, timeline, expectations, and understanding of the proposed arrangement. If you're interviewing the person who will actually provide the care, try to get a sense of how he or she will interact with the elderly person and other family members:

- What experience does the provider have with this type of care?
- How does the provider relate to the elderly person? Does the provider address the elderly person directly and answer his or her questions?
- Are there any cultural, class, or ethnic biases—on either side—that could affect the quality of caregiving?
- Do you and the elderly person understand the provider's answers to your questions?
- Are you comfortable that the relationship can be ended quickly and without penalty if it doesn't work out for any reason?
- Are you clear about the employment relationship? Whom does the provider work for, you or the agency? Is the provider bonded? Does the provider have workers' compensation and malpractice insurance? Who is responsible for finding a substitute if the provider is absent one day? What about night, weekend, vacation, and sick-day coverage?
- Is everyone clear about the services to be provided? This includes the length of time the provider will be needed, the frequency of service, what will happen at each visit, the intended outcome of the service, and the costs involved.
- Does everyone agree on the scope of the services, including whether the provider will perform any other activities or chores?
- Do you sense any communication problems that could arise?

Assess the personality and manner of the potential provider, and make sure that all parties involved understand the arrangement. The importance of clarifying expectations in the contract cannot be overstated. Realistic expectations will help you measure the provider's services, as well as the elderly person's progress. If the goal will be measured in months, don't get upset if the elderly person doesn't show much improvement in the first week.

In some cases, providers will come to the home, provide the service, and leave. In other cases, they will stay in the home for hours at a time—for example, an LPN who provides skilled nursing services to a bedridden elderly person all day. In this case, you need to clarify what the providers will do when they are not actually providing care. While home healthcare aides generally will perform some services that are not care-related, nurses, therapists, and their assistants and technicians generally will not. Expectations need to be worked out in advance. Otherwise, problems can surface when a worker who is being paid a considerable hourly rate spends the afternoon watching soap operas on television.

You may feel like you have to make a hiring decision right away, especially if you're a long-distance caregiver, but remember, this person will be performing a key service in the elderly person's home. It's important to step back, take your time, and choose the best possible service provider.

Hiring the Provider

After you've selected a service provider, it's important to put your understanding in writing. Most agencies will insist on a written contract, but many individual providers will not. Remember, if you work out the details up front and define your expectations in writing, you will minimize problems later on. Do not hesitate to have a professional review the contract, especially if you don't understand everything in it or if it doesn't precisely describe your understanding of the arrangement.

If you think there might be federal, state, and local tax issues, or insurance issues such as worker's compensation, talk to an attorney or insurance consultant before signing anything to be sure you understand what you're committing to. A mistake at this point can be very costly later.

Once a contract has been signed, you must live up to your end of the arrangement, and the provider must live up to his or hers. Monitor the service closely. If the provider is not living up to your understanding of the agreement, question his or her performance as soon as possible.

Occasionally, problems may develop between the provider and the elderly person. If this happens, get involved immediately so you can deal with simple misunderstandings before the relationship is destroyed. If the problem is serious, you may have to replace the provider.

Be as quick to commend good service as you are to question poor performance. Remember, once you involve professional caregivers, caregiving becomes a team effort. To meet the elderly person's needs, there must be communication and respect among all team members.

Caregiving from a Distance

What You Need to Know

Long-distance caregiving is becoming more and more common. While not as physically demanding as traditional caregiving, it is perhaps more stressful because it presents a unique set of challenges.

From a distance, it's almost impossible to get a sense of local resources, not to mention an elderly person's needs. Furthermore, because long-distance caregivers can't provide personal care to the elderly, they must network in the person's community and be as organized as possible when arranging caregiving services. Communication with providers may be difficult, and circumstances can change rapidly. By the time a caregiver is notified of a problem, it may already have evolved into a crisis in need of immediate attention. For these reasons, more and more long-distance caregivers are hiring geriatric care managers (page 189) to coordinate caregiving services.

Hiring a professional can be difficult. In some cases, the services may be too expensive. In others, the elderly person or another family member may oppose the notion of outsiders providing care. If the elderly person has no pressing medical problems and seems to be muddling along, the family may not understand why a geriatric care manager is needed. Where money isn't an issue, however, families are likely to support the idea if the elderly person's need for assistance becomes more obvious.

To get the names of care managers in the elderly person's community, contact the National Association of Professional Geriatric Care Managers listed in chapter 7, or simply look in the phone book. Make some phone calls and set up interviews for your next visit.

Never hire a professional over the phone, except in an extreme emergency or when an interview is impossible (see Choosing Professionals beginning on page 189). In an emergency, you may have to hire a geriatric care manager to help with the immediate problem, but be sure to evaluate his or her performance before making a long-term arrangement.

Finding Local Resources
Phone Books

Even if you hire a caregiving coordinator, be sure to have a local telephone book so you can contact individuals or organizations in the elderly person's community. While the *Telephone Contact Lists* in chapter 7 will provide many key phone numbers, a local phone book can be indispensable when you're not exactly sure whom to call. Let's say you want to arrange for meals to be delivered to the elderly person's home, but the Meals-on-Wheels program has a different name in his or her community. When you don't know whom to contact or what services are available, the local telephone book, with its full-page ads, is a good place to start. Be sure to get copies of the White, Blue, and Yellow Pages.

Hospital Discharge Planners

If the elderly person is admitted to the hospital and will need ongoing medical or nursing services after he or she is discharged, the hospital discharge planner will prepare a care plan. He or she can also help arrange the necessary home healthcare services. If you like the hospital discharge planner with whom you're working, consider hiring him or her to advise you in future emergencies that do not involve a hospital visit.

Area Agency on Aging

If the elderly person hasn't been admitted to a hospital, his or her local Area Agency on Aging may be a good source of free information. The staff should be knowledgeable about community resources. While these agencies won't make contacts for you or research options the way a hospital discharge planner will, they can point you in the right direction. These agencies may also be listed in the phone book under Senior Citizen's Information Center or Mayor's Office on Aging.

Other Resources

Other free resources that are invaluable to all caregivers include the following:
- The United Way
- The Red Cross
- The American Association of Retired Persons (AARP)

- Hospital supply companies (for information about assistive devices)
- The Visiting Nurses Association
- Meals-on-Wheels
- Medicare or Medicaid helplines
- The Legal Aid Society
- Churches or synagogues
- Eldercare Locator: 1-800-677-1116 (they will ask for the elderly person's name, address, and a description of his or her problem)
- Home healthcare agencies (their services aren't free, but you can call them for information about costs and services available)
- Organizations and associations for specific diseases or illnesses (see chapter 7)
- Local support groups
- The public library's help or information desk
- The Internet (many Internet sites have links to local organizations—see chapter 7)

Visiting the Elderly

It can be difficult to coordinate in-home services by telephone, fax, or mail. While you can rely on these to some extent, it's essential to periodically visit the elderly person so you can observe his or her needs firsthand. Each visit is an opportunity to assess the elderly person's situation, network in the community, and lay the groundwork for future caregiving decisions.

Fact-finding and decision-making visits can be quite stressful for the elderly. These visits—which never seem to be long enough—carry a sense of urgency for long-distance caregivers. After all, caregivers need to use every minute wisely and make decisions quickly. This can create a sense of panic in the elderly, particularly if caregiving decisions are made without their involvement. As difficult as it may sound, it's important to include the elderly person whenever possible and to try to project a sense of calm when visiting, gathering information, and making caregiving decisions. This will make the process less stressful for both of you.

Assessing the Situation

Before your visit, try to get a clear idea of the elderly person's living conditions; physical, mental, emotional, and financial status; and healthcare, home care, and housekeeping needs. The elderly person, his or her friends, local caregivers, and your community network can all help you get this information.

Once you arrive in the elderly person's home, review the home safety section (page 79) and Assessing the Risk of Living at Home (page 96) to evaluate the elderly person's living conditions. The *Activities of Daily Living Checklist* (page 77) and the *Home Care and Housekeeping Form* (page 109) will help you assess his or her needs. For every need, think of a backup plan. Ask yourself, How will we meet this need if something breaks, if the weather is bad, or if the service provider doesn't show up? It isn't easy to think of all the things that could go wrong, but by considering the possibilities, discussing potential problems with others, and making a phone call or two, you'll be better prepared to handle most problems as they arise.

Networking in the Community
Meeting Professionals

Set an agenda for your visit. List everything you hope to accomplish and everyone you wish to speak with. Plan on making the most efficient use of your time. If you know you want to meet with specific professionals, agencies, support groups, friends, or community services, call in advance to schedule appointments. If possible, have the other people come to meet you. That way, you can be sure there will be no interruptions, and you won't waste time driving around, looking for parking, or waiting. If you intend to hire a service provider who will interact with the elderly person, try to arrange interviews so that the elderly person can participate.

If you hire a professional or engage a service during your visit, have the person or service start before you leave so you can take care of any problems that may arise. Don't assist; simply observe how well the service will work when you're not there. (See also Selecting In-Home Care Providers on page 111.)

Meeting Friends and Acquaintances

In addition to meeting all caregivers (paid and volunteer), get to know acquaintances of the elderly— their friends, where they shop, who does their hair, who they call or see regularly, where they worship, and who visits them. Get names and telephone numbers whenever possible. If something comes up, you may need to contact one of these people for more information or for help in an emergency. Also, if any of these people do something to help the elderly person, you should recognize their contribution by sending a thank-you card or gift with a personal note.

Most importantly, when you meet the elderly person's friends and acquaintances, give them your name and phone number and encourage them to contact you if anything goes wrong. In fact, you may want to hand out an emergency contact list (see chapter 7) that tells them how to get in touch with you, other family members, the person's geriatric care manager, the person's doctor, and anyone else who should be contacted in an emergency. You may also want to leave an extra house key with a trusted neighbor.

Preparing for Future Caregiving Decisions

Now is the time to collect information about the elderly person's financial position, medical history, medications, and living condition, as well as his or her physical, mental, and emotional condition. If you have the time, fill out the following forms:

- *Vital Information Form* (pages 9–33)
- *Financial Worksheets* (pages 39–54)
- *Basic Medical Information* (pages 57–61)
- *Medication List* (pages 70–72)
- *Document Collection Form* (pages 197–213)
- *Telephone Contact Lists* (pages 214–224)

Be sure to evaluate the elderly person's home (page 79) during your visit. You might also discuss advance directives and fill out a *Values History Form* (page 177). Together, you and the elderly person can talk about how his or her needs will be met and start thinking about backup plans in case something goes wrong.

Emergency Planning

As a long-distance caregiver, you should have a plan for emergencies. Otherwise, if an emergency arises, you'll have no idea where to begin, whom to contact, or what to do until you get to the elderly person's home. If, however, you've started to develop a local network that you can call on in a crisis, you'll be able to begin dealing with the situation right away. A few phone calls before you arrive will help you to hit the ground running once you get there.

Talk to the elderly person about what needs to be done in an emergency (for example, if he or she is suddenly admitted to the hospital) and record all the relevant phone numbers on the *Caregiver Emergency Contact List* on page 217. You may need to know the following:

- Which newspapers to stop
- How to handle the mail and any pets
- Whom to contact to water the plants and remove perishable food from the refrigerator
- What home care or housekeeping services to call
- Whether you need to notify a telephone reassurance service (see page 103)
- Whom the elderly person wants you to contact

If a crisis occurs, you won't be able to do much until you arrive. However, with your emergency contact list, you'll be able to take care of some of the more immediate issues before you leave home.

Chapter 5

Alternative Housing Options

At one time, elderly people who could no longer live alone basically had two options: they could either live in a nursing home or move into someone's house, usually a relative's. In the last twenty years, however, there's been an explosion in housing alternatives. New housing opportunities are constantly being created, and there's no reason to think that this won't accelerate in the years ahead. Nevertheless, the elderly often view housing issues from the limited perspective of what was available when they were concerned about their parents. They may fear moving from their home because they don't want to be stuck in a nursing home. Although a nursing home is only one of many housing options, the elderly frequently reject all other alternatives without further exploration.

Many caregivers are also unaware of elder housing alternatives in their community. As a result, both an elderly person and his or her family may go to extreme lengths to keep that person in his or her home, even though another housing option would be safer and more appropriate.

Exploring the Choices

What You Need to Know

Although the elderly may prefer to remain at home, many circumstances could cause the elderly to move unexpectedly. There are three main issues that might force you to confront the question of alternative housing:

1. Maintaining the home becomes too much of a physical, mental, emotional, or financial burden for the elderly person or his or her caregivers.

2. Outside circumstances significantly affect the person's home or care. For example, the lease expires, the primary caregiver is unable to continue providing assistance, or the home is damaged by a storm.

3. A change in the elderly person's condition makes the home unsafe or unsuitable. For example, worsening dementia, an inability to climb stairs, or an inability to get necessities.

Although you may not face any of these circumstances now, advance planning will prepare you to deal with unexpected or sudden changes when they occur. Furthermore, many housing options have eligibility requirements, and the most desirable facilities are likely to have waiting lists. Failing to plan ahead may necessitate having to move the elderly person several times before the desired facility becomes available, which can be traumatic for everyone involved, especially the elderly person.

Continuum of Care

When comparing housing alternatives, you'll often see the term "continuum of care" in advertising and promotional materials. "Continuum of care" can mean many different things, but it basically indicates that a range of living arrangements are available. It's important to find out what these options are and how they might be paid for. If a company says they cover the "continuum of care," they may mean any of the following:

• They offer living arrangements such as senior condominiums or apartments with an acute care hospital or long-term care facility nearby. Note: the cost of these services is not necessarily included. The company may provide the services, or they might contract some of them out to another provider. Also, they may not provide all the levels of care that you might expect in a continuum. For example, they might offer a basic assisted-living facility for $2,500 per month, but the next level of care might be a nursing home at $4,500 per month. A level of care somewhere between these two options—such as an assisted-living facility that provides a high level of custodial care for $3,250 a month—may not be available.

• As the elderly person's needs change, he or she automatically will be moved (or have the right to move) from one level of housing to another within the system. The integrated system is in place and is being paid for by the elderly person, the life care community (see page 122), or Medicaid. In this case, it's important to find out who decides if the level of care must be changed and what your appeal rights are.

• They offer a managed care arrangement. In this case, an insurer or government agency is paying the provider a set amount to provide services, which may include housing and nursing services, to the elderly person. How much and what type of care is provided is left up to the provider, and the insured person has little say in the process. This is basically an extension of the HMO model of healthcare to housing.

Housing Options Summarized

For ease of explanation, the following housing alternatives have been somewhat arbitrarily divided into two major categories: independent housing and residential housing. Each category contains two or three general housing options, and each option offers several possible living arrangements. While the precise name for each type of housing varies from place to place, if you focus on the characteristics, you can determine what that type of housing is called in your community. These living arrangements are discussed in greater detail beginning on page 121.

Independent Housing
Nonsubsidized senior housing
- Senior adult condominiums
- Continuing care retirement communities (CCRCs)
- Life care communities
- Senior apartments
- Senior retirement centers
- Retirement hotels

Subsidized senior housing
- Section 202 housing
- Public housing
- Subsidized congregate housing
- Supported housing for seniors with disabilities

Shared housing
- Eldercare housing opportunity (ECHO)
- Small group housing
- Adult foster care
- Matched housing

Residential housing
Assisted-living housing
- Assisted-living facilities
- Personal care homes
- Board-and-care facilities
- Specialty personal care homes

Healthcare-related housing
- Extended care hospital
- Stepdown or sub-acute unit
- Rehabilitation facilities
- Rest homes
- Convalescent homes
- Homes for the aged
- Nursing homes
- Hospice care

It can be difficult to find out which kinds of housing are available in your community, especially when you encounter meaningless or confusing names like Golden Pond or Amber Mountain: Personal Care for the Independent Senior. There's no way of knowing with certainty what the five main housing alternatives are called in your community, or whether a facility of each type even exists. However, ads in the Yellow Pages and healthcare publications may offer at least a partial description of local facilities, and geriatric care managers and discharge planners can be an excellent source of information.

Independent Housing

In general, independent housing is only available to elderly people who are basically healthy and independent, and who have no major difficulties with any of the Activities of Daily Living (page 77). Be wary of entering into a long-term contract, however, because a sudden change in health may require a move to a new living facility on short notice.

With any independent housing arrangement, it is important to maintain regular contact with the elderly person. However, group housing, adult foster care, and matched housing represent a significant loss of privacy and may expose the elderly to abuse and neglect by housemates and unlicensed caregivers. If the elderly person has chosen one of these housing options, it's especially important to check his or her status through visits and telephone calls.

Nonsubsidized Senior Housing
Senior Adult Condominiums

With this option, the elderly person owns the unit. Condominium complexes can range from 20 to 150 units, from expensive to moderately priced. Maintenance fees on condominiums, which can be costly, cover maintenance, security, and some social and recreational services. They generally have a minimum age for ownership (usually age fifty-five), and residents must hire any personal or medical services on their own. Because senior condominiums are almost like living alone, they are best compared to home ownership rather than other kinds of senior housing. Any regulation is provided by the resident-controlled condominium association.

Senior adult condominiums have several advantages: the size and style of the condominium can be matched to the person's lifestyle, needs, and interests; the person can keep his or her possessions; the person will be surrounded by elderly companions; and transportation to shopping and malls is readily available. In addition, there are many opportunities for recreation, socializing, and participation in the condominium government.

There are few maintenance or security concerns, and in-home services are usually easy to arrange.

The disadvantages may include restrictive rules, especially when it comes to visits by grandchildren. Fees can be high and may be affected by events beyond the elderly person's control. If the person is forced to leave, he or she is obligated to pay maintenance fees and taxes until the unit is sold, although some nonprofit and religious organizations may purchase the unit if it isn't sold within a specified period of time. While services may be easy to arrange, most caregiving needs and problems are still an issue. Finally, when other owners move or die, the elderly person may not like the newcomers.

Continuing Care Retirement Communities (CCRCs)

CCRCs, also called life care communities, are licensed by the state and offer independent living, either as part of a large complex (which might include an apartment unit, an assisted-living facility, and a nursing home), or as a separate apartment building associated with a nearby assisted-living facility and nursing home. The choice of a unified complex or a separate facility is usually based on space considerations or philosophical beliefs; it is unrelated to the quality of care. The apartments are rarely furnished.

Most communities have a costly entrance fee, along with a monthly fee that covers rent, some meals, housekeeping, security, social and recreational programs, and limited transportation. In addition to these services, the community may agree to provide housing, medical care, or support needed for the rest of the elderly person's life.

Although there are many CCRCs around the country, they're not always a viable option. Many are selective in who they will admit, and the entrance fee may cost hundreds of thousands of dollars. However, their services are almost always first-rate and often can be negotiated upon admittance.

If this is what the elderly person wants and can afford, it should remove most housing, healthcare, and home care concerns.

A significant issue is the financial strength of the life care contract provider. Although CCRCs and life care communities are regulated entities, if they don't have a strong financial position, there's always a risk that they may file for bankruptcy or breach their commitment to lifelong care. Elderly who have spent their entire savings on a CCRC entrance fee could end up destitute and homeless, just when their need for caregiving is the greatest. Don't be misled by the impressive surroundings or what you are told. Check references, accreditation, and the length of time the CCRC has been in operation, and be sure to hire a professional to research the company's financial status.

With the rise of managed care, CCRCs are likely to become more common because they allow providers and third-party insurers to control the quality and cost of care. As a result, these programs may be offered to the very poor, since state Medicaid programs will likely contract with managed care providers to provide a continuum of care. From Medicaid's perspective, dealing with one provider that offers a range of services is better than paying many different providers, as it does now.

Senior Apartments and Senior Retirement Centers

These options differ from senior condominiums in two respects. First, they are rental units. The elderly have privacy and are able to select a unit that fits their needs. Although there is a lease, the elderly don't have to deal with the hassle of selling the unit if they move. Second, these units often come with some level of support—property management, maintenance, security, transportation, home care services, recreation, and meals in a common dining area. There usually isn't an entrance fee, although there may be a fee to get on the waiting list.

Although senior apartments and senior retirement centers aren't considered subsidized housing, some communities set limits on personal income. You may also have to show that the elderly person can function safely and independently in an apartment. Generally, personal services, such as the monitoring of medication, are not available (although you can hire a companion). These units normally don't contract with other providers, and they have virtually no state regulation.

Retirement Hotels

Most retirement hotels offer a single room with a private or semi-private bathroom. The rooms may or may not be furnished, and there is regular, if not daily, maid service. For an additional fee, you can get meals in a common dining room. Other than maintenance and security, few services are provided.

Subsidized Senior Housing
Section 202 Housing, Public Housing, and Subsidized Congregate Housing

Each of these is a form of government-subsidized housing; they're only available to elderly people with limited financial resources. Although these apartments tend to be in large, sterile complexes, they almost always have a waiting list because they're the one housing alternative that almost everyone can afford. To get on a list, the elderly person normally must meet specific age, income, and physical independence criteria.

The cost of subsidized senior housing includes maintenance and limited security. Certain services, such as meals, may be purchased, and some buildings offer social and recreational activities. It's usually easy to hire home and personal care services. For more information on these options, contact your local housing authority or Department of Housing and Urban Development (HUD) office.

Supported Housing for Seniors with Disabilities

Supported housing is relatively new. There are few facilities, and these have long waiting lists. The units are designed to accommodate adults with chronic physical or mental disabilities. Maintenance, security, recreation, and sometimes limited meal service are covered, but transportation, laundry, shopping, and home care services will involve an additional expense. Usually, facilitators or social workers will help coordinate the services needed to accommodate specific disabilities. Because this type of facility mixes physically and mentally disabled people, supported housing can be a difficult transition for a person who has only recently become disabled.

The cost of supported housing is often partly underwritten by nonprofit organizations and churches rather than government agencies. When it isn't underwritten, it can be relatively expensive because it is so specialized. In this case, it isn't really subsidized housing, but elderly people with low or moderate incomes may qualify for federal or state support. Many of the organizations listed in chapter 7 can provide information about local housing programs and financial assistance for individuals with certain chronic conditions.

Shared Housing
Eldercare Housing Opportunity (ECHO)

An Australian concept, ECHO actually involves shared land rather than shared housing. The family purchases a small, cottage-like home or trailer that is architecturally similar to the main residence and places it on their property. This way, both the elderly person and the family maintain their privacy and independence, but help is nearby. This alternative may be problematic in areas with land-use planning, building codes, and zoning.

Small Group Housing

This is what most people think of as shared housing. A group of people, from four to twenty, live in a large home or converted building, usually under the auspices of a church or nonprofit group. They pay monthly rent, live together, and do some work around the house. The rent and other arrangements vary depending on the services provided. In some group homes, residents are self-sufficient; in others, everything is provided for them. The larger the group, the more likely it is that there will be a live-in social worker or manager to organize things and deal with the issues that invariably arise when a group of people live in such proximity. Financial assistance is available in some cases.

Adult Foster Care

Here, an elderly person or couple moves in with a person who provides room and board, basic personal care, and housekeeping services. Although this service can be arranged privately or through a nonprofit organization, social service agencies often make these placements and follow up to be sure the elderly person is healthy and receiving the care he or she needs.

Matched Housing

Here, someone moves in with an elderly person who has no major caregiving needs. Arrangements like these are usually made privately. In exchange for free room and board and a monthly stipend, the elderly person has a live-in companion—a friend, college student, or young relative—who runs errands, provides home care, and may assist with the Activities of Daily Living. If no caregiving services are expected and the live-in person is just there in case of an emergency, this individual may even pay rent.

Residential Housing

The housing options that follow offer care in a residential setting. They provide personal care and/or medical services based on the elderly person's needs.

Assisted-Living Housing
Assisted-Living Facilities, Personal Care Homes, and Board-and-Care Facilities

In some states, assisted-living facilities are licensed by the Department of Social Services or its equivalent. In states where they're not licensed, employees of these facilities don't provide healthcare services. All facilities must meet minimum standards, and there's usually some kind of monitoring to ensure compliance. Government oversight of assisted-living homes, however, is generally much less rigorous than that of nursing homes.

Assisted-living facilities are one step away from living independently. They offer a private, safe, and comfortable environment, and most residents are mobile and able to handle most of their physical needs. The rooms range from fairly luxurious private rooms or small apartments to semi-private rooms in an institutional setting. Laundry, maintenance, security, transportation, recreation, doctor and clergy visits, communal meals, housekeeping, medication management, and twenty-four-hour monitoring are routinely provided. In some states, these services can be negotiated and paid for separately.

Even with monthly charges around $1,500 to $3,000, assisted-living facilities can be quite cost-effective because they can meet all personal care needs except skilled nursing services. Generally, neither Medicare nor Medicaid will cover the basic monthly charge; almost all residents pay privately. Low-income, blind, or disabled residents may be able to pay by combining state welfare payments and Supplemental Security Income (SSI) payments. Long-term care insurance might cover the basic monthly charge, depending on the person's condition and the terms of the policy.

Assisted-living facilities may be an excellent alternative for elderly people who are unable to live alone but don't need healthcare or nursing services. However, if this is the elderly person's first admission to a residential setting, be careful to include him or her in the selection process as much as possible. While adjusting to their new living arrangement, the elderly may feel helpless and resent their loss of privacy. They may rebel, become depressed, express feelings of abandonment, and even attempt to wander away.

When selecting an assisted-living facility, consider the issues covered in the *Residential Housing Form* beginning on page 155. Although an assisted-living facility is a viable option when independent living is no longer safe, you need to realistically consider the elderly person's needs. Assisted-living isn't appropriate for a person with serious mental or emotional problems, such as severe dementia. You should also note that more and more assisted-living facilities are admitting (or keeping) residents who need services and care that they cannot provide. This dangerous situation exists because of the lack of effective regulation, and because caregivers don't know what level of care to expect.

Specialty Personal Care Homes

In many communities, specialty personal care homes have evolved to deal with special needs, such as AIDS and Alzheimer's disease. These facilities tend to be more expensive than regular assisted-living facilities, but if there's a facility in the community that offers the kind of care the elderly person requires, it's worth considering.

Generally, all the services normally offered in an assisted-living facility are available in a specialty personal care home, but the staff is more highly trained and motivated.

These homes often have specially designed programs and support groups for residents and their caregivers. In Alzheimer's facilities, the patients live in a secure building, and much attention may have gone into the facility's design, decoration, and staffing to calm the patients and help them adjust to their surroundings. Sometimes a facility offers an Alzheimer's daycare unit or respite care for caregivers. In AIDS facilities, there may be an emphasis on nursing, counseling, and hospice care.

Be careful about committing an elderly person to a specialized facility or a more expensive unit within an existing facility. In some cases, nothing will be especially unique about the facility, the unit, or the staff. The only things that may be different are the name and the fee. Before admitting the person to a special unit, talk with local support groups, doctors, discharge planners, and geriatric care managers. Also, be sure to check all references, especially families of existing residents.

Healthcare-Related Housing
Extended Care Hospital

As managed care and healthcare cost-containment programs continue to have a negative impact on hospital admissions, some acute care hospitals are converting either partially or entirely to extended care hospitals. These provide care to individuals with chronic medical conditions or diseases that do not require admission to an acute care hospital. They generally provide the same type and level of care that is offered in high-quality nursing homes or rehabilitation hospitals. Most of the services are covered by insurance, Medicaid, and sometimes Medicare.

Stepdown or Sub-Acute Unit

The stepdown or sub-acute unit of an acute care hospital houses patients who need skilled nursing care or therapy but can no longer be justified as an acute care admission. Many Medicare-certified nursing homes also have sub-acute units. These units are designed for short stays, measured in days or weeks, and the services are almost always covered by Medicare or insurance.

Medicare places a limit on the number of days it will cover skilled nursing care in a person's lifetime. Days spent in a stepdown or sub-acute unit are counted against this lifetime limit. When insurance or Medicare coverage ends, hospital patients are usually discharged to their home or a nursing home. Nursing home patients, however, may qualify for Medicaid. If they don't, they must pay for their care privately.

Rehabilitation Facilities

Most of the services provided in a stepdown or sub-acute unit can also be provided in a rehabilitation hospital, institute, or clinic. However, rehabilitation hospitals tend to provide these services more intensively, on a short-term basis, and with an emphasis on physical or occupational therapy. Most rehabilitation patients come from an acute care hospital, and their stay is measured in days or weeks rather than months or years. Because of the nature of the services provided, they are covered by Medicare and insurance.

Rehabilitation facilities may be considered a kind of temporary housing. This option is often overlooked after a hospital stay. Rehabilitation facilities provide intensive therapy designed to strengthen the patient and train both patient and caregiver so the person will be able to live as safely as possible at home. Rehabilitation therapists are quite knowledgeable about assistive devices; they may visit the person's home to suggest modifications that will make the home safer and more accessible.

Rest Homes, Convalescent Homes, and Homes for the Aged

In some states, rest homes, convalescent homes, and homes for the aged are similar to assisted-living facilities. In other states they're like nursing homes, except they lack the more specialized and intensive medical options that many urban nursing homes have.

These homes are licensed facilities, often in rural areas, that rely on Medicaid and private payments. They provide an intermediate level of care: some nursing care is available, but residents are usually fairly mobile and self-sufficient. The homes offer meals, social services, and twenty-four-hour medical and personal care, usually in a setting with less than fifty beds.

Nursing Homes and Long-Term Care Facilities

The last two decades have seen a dramatic shift in the services provided by state-licensed nursing homes, who lives in these homes, and how the services are paid for. Today, nursing homes offer the same sub-acute, rehabilitation, and specialty services that are offered in extended care hospitals, rehabilitation hospitals, or stepdown or sub-acute units. Medicare and managed care insurers are discovering that the same treatment results can be achieved as efficiently in nursing homes as in these other facilities.

Most people think of a nursing home as an elderly person's permanent residence for the rest of his or her life. But two key services—rehabilitation and sub-acute care—are short-term in nature. Patients who are discharged from a hospital are likely to be admitted to a nursing home for this type of care. They may stay for several days or weeks and then go home. Whether short-term or long-term, all nursing home residents have a mental or physical impairment that prevents them from living independently and is severe enough that an assisted-living facility cannot provide the necessary care.

Unfortunately, quality of care is a concern among nursing home residents and their families. When selecting a nursing home, caregivers must carefully consider a variety of factors, but perhaps none is so critical as the quality of care, which is discussed in detail on page 146.

Hospice Care

Hospice care can be supplied in one of several settings—at home, in a hospice, or in a nursing home. Usually, the elderly person is dying or is only expected to live a short time. Hospice care is an alternative to the aggressive medical approach that is meant to keep a person alive without regard to his or her quality of life. It is usually paid for by Medicare, Medicaid, or insurance. If the elderly person wants hospice care but does not qualify under one of these programs, ask for an exception. Exceptions are routinely granted by third-party payers, because hospice care is far cheaper than any of the alternatives.

Moving In with the Caregiver

The obvious option that hasn't been discussed so far is to move the elderly person in with the caregiver or another family member. This is almost always a mistake. It is very hard to provide the nursing and personal care that an elderly person needs 24 hours a day, 7 days a week, 365 days a year. Even if the elderly person is mentally alert, self-sufficient, and mobile, this option should never be chosen without careful consideration of what it will involve.

Before you proceed, thoroughly discuss the following issues—and any others that are unique to your situation—with everyone involved. If you're not comfortable with, or in complete agreement on, all of these points, you should be cautious about having the elderly person move in with you.

1. Will the move be temporary or permanent? A temporary move can take many different forms. The person may move in until he or she recovers from an accident, with the understanding that he or she will move out in the near future. The move could be a temporary arrangement until another form of housing becomes available. Or, the elderly person's stay could be open-ended, with the understanding that he or she will move to more appropriate housing when his or her physical health warrants it. Whatever the arrangement, don't assume that the elderly person understands—you need to specifically discuss the move with him or her, as well as with other family members. Otherwise, when the next move becomes necessary, somebody may feel betrayed or misled.

2. What will happen to the elderly person's possessions? Even if you believe the move will be permanent, it may be wise to keep the elderly person's home and furnishings for a while. If the move doesn't work out, and you have already disposed of the elderly person's possessions, this might limit his or her housing alternatives.

3. Is there adequate space? This question is one of the most important. Using the extra bedroom is not an adequate answer. Regardless of the elderly person's physical and mental condition, having another person in the house will affect more than a single room. You need to consider bathroom use, kitchen safety, incontinence, room temperature, visitors, activity and noise level, telephone use, pets, and privacy. Consider these issues not only from the standpoint of the elderly person, but also from the perspective of others in the household.

4. Will caregiving require in-home services by outsiders? When considering how the household will be affected, don't overlook the accommodations that will have to be made for professional caregivers. If home healthcare aides or therapists will be coming into the home regularly, consider how this will affect the privacy and convenience of other household members, including children.

5. What physical changes will need to be made to your home? Refer to the *Home Safety Checklists* beginning on page 81 to see how to make a home safe for the elderly. Use these lists to determine what changes you will need to make to your home. Then ask yourself: "Do I want to make the necessary changes? Can I afford to make them? How will these changes affect other household members? Will these changes have to be permanent? If so, how will they affect the resale value of my home?"

6. Will this new living arrangement increase the level of stress in the household? Few households are completely free of stress. While long-distance caregiving is stressful, having someone move into your home may be more stressful. Consider whether everyone will be able to get along, day after day. Conflicts that already exist are likely to get worse with daily contact. Lastly, consider whether the move will create a precedent for other elderly relatives. If you do this for your parent(s), will you be expected to do it for your spouse's parent(s) as well?

7. Do you feel pressured to have the elderly person move in? Is guilt or concern about what others will think a major factor in your decision? Is your decision voluntary? If the answer isn't an unequivocal "yes" for all parties involved, you need to confront this before you make your decision. If the elderly person moves in and you haven't honestly addressed these issues, feelings of resentment, anger, and hostility are likely to build over time.

8. What sacrifices will you or the elderly person have to make? Caregiving costs money, in terms of both the care you provide and the money you can't earn outside the home while you're providing this care. If you're currently working, you should seriously consider if the new arrangement will force you to cut back your hours. Also consider if reducing your hours, being forced to take an unpaid leave of absence, or missing work because an outside caregiver fails to show up could reduce your chances of advancement or even cost you your job.

From the elderly person's standpoint, moving may mean giving up an active social life. The person may be moving away from friends, church, and volunteer work—all the social activities that connect him or her to a community. Completely severing these ties may have serious consequences, including depression. While any move will cause this to happen to some extent, many housing options offer a community of other elderly people and opportunities to socialize.

Although this discussion may sound overly pessimistic, the fact is that we no longer live in the era of the extended family, where families live in proximity and grow old together. Today's single-parent families and working couples must carefully consider all the issues before introducing another person into their household. If everyone, including the elderly person, understands exactly what obligations are involved and what the limits of those obligations will be, this will reduce the likelihood of problems in the future.

While this is an area of real anxiety for many caregivers, feelings of guilt or obligation should not outweigh a rational assessment of the responsibility you'd be undertaking—and how it would affect the elderly person, yourself, and your family. If your circumstances permit it, having the elderly person move in can be an excellent solution to the housing issue. However, this is a serious commitment that should not be undertaken lightly, since caregiving mistakes can lead to the injury or even death of the elderly person. Assess this option as you would any other housing alternative to find the best way to meet the elderly person's needs.

Choosing Appropriate Housing

What You Need to Know

Although choosing housing for an elderly person can be a long and difficult process, in some cases, the decision will be made for you. A physician might order or prescribe a particular rehabilitation hospital, or the elderly person may decide that he or she wants to live in a particular assisted-living facility. If his or her needs can be met and finances are not an issue, you can focus on arranging the move and monitoring the quality and appropriateness of the elderly person's care.

It is far more likely, however, that you will be intimately involved in any housing decision. Caregivers often must act as scouts and fact gatherers, framing the issues for the elderly and their families so that the best decision will be made. In many cases, caregivers are the ones to make the actual decision.

The rest of this chapter will help you focus on finding the most appropriate housing in your community. It addresses a number of questions and issues that need to be considered during the selection process. Certain alternatives are not discussed, such as rehabilitation hospitals, since admission to this kind of facility is usually ordered by a doctor. Likewise, the decision to go to a hospice reflects a preference about how life should end rather than how it should be lived.

The distinctions between independent and residential housing are merely to help explain the range of alternatives. When you begin looking at housing options, do not focus on finding a type of housing that has the same name used in this chapter. For example, the term "matched housing" may not exist in your community—in fact, local professionals may not even have heard of it—and terms like "personal care" will mean different things in different communities. Simply look for housing that the elderly person can afford and qualify for, and that can best address his or her needs.

An easy way to start is to refer back to the *Home Care and Housekeeping Form* (page 109) and *Activities of Daily Living Checklist* (page 77) to identify the elderly person's problems or needs. The following are examples of some of the most common problems that the elderly face, along with suggestions for appropriate housing.

PROBLEM: Need significant, but short-term, care.
APPROPRIATE HOUSING: (1) Temporary residential housing, such as a nursing home or rehabilitation facility. (2) Remain at home and hire a home healthcare service.

PROBLEM: Need significant long-term care.
APPROPRIATE HOUSING: Residential housing, such as an assisted-living or convalescent home.

PROBLEM: Living at home is increasingly difficult because of frailty or medical problems.
APPROPRIATE HOUSING: Residential housing, such as a home for the aged or a nursing home.

PROBLEM: Not enough money to continue maintaining home.
APPROPRIATE HOUSING: Independent housing, such as shared housing or subsidized senior housing

How to Use the *Housing Selection Form*

The following worksheet will help you narrow your housing options based on the elderly person's needs, the housing alternatives in your community, the financial resources available, and whether the elderly person is eligible for certain facilities.

In the first section, list the elderly person's needs. Be as specific as possible. You may wish to refer to the *Home Care and Housekeeping Form* (page 109) and the *Activities of Daily Living Checklist* (page 77) when filling out this section. Remember, you are looking for appropriate housing, so the most serious need will almost always determine the most appropriate alternative. For example, occasional violent outbursts could rule out an assisted-living facility, even if assisted living could meet the rest of the elderly person's needs.

In the second section, list the type of housing that you and the elderly person believe to be most appropriate. Refer to the descriptions of housing alternatives on pages 121–127 for assistance.

In the third section, summarize the eligibility requirements for the housing option selected and whether or not the elderly person can afford it. This may require a bit of research on your part, such as a visit to that kind of housing facility or a discussion with a social worker. (You may also need to refer to the *Financial Worksheets* on pages 39–54.)

In the last section, identify specific facilities in your community for the type of housing selected. List only those facilities that (1) meet the elderly person's needs, (2) the elderly person can afford, and (3) the elderly person is eligible for.

HOUSING SELECTION FORM

Needs/level of independence _____

_____

_____

_____

_____

_____

_____

_____

Appropriate housing _____

_____

_____

_____

_____

Cost/eligibility requirements_____

_____

_____

_____

_____

Facilities available _____

_____

_____

_____

_____

_____

_____

A Family Caregiver's Guide to Planning and Decision Making for the Elderly © 1999 James A. Wilkinson

How to Find Independent Housing

What You Need to Know

By definition, independent housing is for relatively independent people, and independent people should be involved in the housing selection process as much as possible. They may have friends or acquaintances living in a particular facility, and they might express an interest in moving there if a move becomes necessary. If the facility can meet their needs and a space is (or soon will be) available, the selection process can be relatively easy.

If the elderly person shows no preference toward a particular facility, or if it isn't clear which alternative is the best, you'll need to identify different housing options on your own. If there are no openings in the facility you prefer, you'll need to find a short-term arrangement until space opens up. If your first choice isn't available, it's best to look for the next-highest level of care—that is, housing with services that are slightly more intensive than the person needs. It makes more sense to move to a facility where the elderly person doesn't need all of the services offered than to a facility that can't meet the person's existing needs, let alone future needs. The elderly person may not like this alternative, however, and he or she should have a say in the decision.

Once you have identified several potential facilities, you and the elderly person should visit them together. Before the visit, get as many different opinions about the facility as you can. Start with the elderly person's friends (especially any who live at the facility), the local Area Agency on Aging, a hospital discharge planner, the Better Business Bureau, the elderly person's doctor, and even a clergy member in the community. These conversations should give you a feel for the facility's reputation and quality, and they may raise issues or concerns that you'll want to address during your visit.

Because independent living facilities offer a private living space, tour the spaces that are available, not just the models. Check them thoroughly and make sure everything works—the lights, appliances, windows and doors, locks, and so forth. For a CCRC or any other facility offering continuum of care, tour the space where the person would live, then tour the next-highest level of care (use the *Residential Housing Form* beginning on page 155), even if it doesn't seem relevant now.

You should also review the facility's promotional material (the official explanation of why the elderly person would want to live there). Work your network to find out if the services are being delivered appropriately or if any problems exist, and don't hesitate to ask a financial planner or elderlaw attorney to review contracts, leases, and financial statements. Check references whenever possible, and be especially sensitive about situations that don't feel right.

How to Use the *Independent Housing Form*

The *Independent Housing Form* will help you gather the information you need to compare different housing facilities. You can use it to determine what services are included in the housing, what they will cost, and how you'll be able to get out of the obligation when the time comes. You'll need to make several copies of this form and fill out one for each location you visit. You might also wish to tailor the list of questions to fit your specific needs.

INDEPENDENT HOUSING FORM

Basic Information

Facility name_____

Address _____

Telephone number_____

Fax number_____

Manager or contact person _____

May we have a copy of the admission package (financial information, rules and regulations, brochures)? _____

May we have copies of the legal documents necessary for admission?

_____

Is there a vacancy? _____

Is there a waiting list? How long until an opening is expected?

_____

Is there a fee or deposit to get on the waiting list? Is it refundable?

_____

What if we don't take the first available vacancy?

_____

Admission and Financial Information

What are the admission criteria? _____

_____

Is a doctor's statement required? (usually about the person's ability to perform Activities of Daily Living—see page 76) _____

_____

Do we need evidence of the elderly person's age, income, assets, or ability to pay? _____

_____

For a shared living arrangement, do residents have any say in roommate selection? What if the new resident doesn't work out or can't adjust?

_____

What is the monthly fee? What is included in the monthly fee?

_____

What services can the person expect to be billed for that aren't included in the basic monthly fee (transportation, nonroutine maintenance, recreation, outings, laundry, housekeeping, meals, and so forth)?

_____

Is there a fee schedule? _____

How often do fees increase? When was the last increase?

_____

When are charges billed? _____

Are charges itemized? _____

When are charges due? _____

Is there a penalty for late payment? _____

What happens if a payment is missed? Who is notified? _____

_____

If there's a problem with the bill, who must be notified and by when?

_____

Are security deposits or advance payments required? _____

Are deposits refundable? On what terms? _____

Are there extra charges for installing telephones, televisions, and so forth? Are there ongoing monthly fees? _____

_____

If the person is admitted to a hospital, what ongoing fees will he or she be responsible for? _____

_____

For subsidized housing: What happens if the eligibility criteria are no longer met? _____

_____

For shared housing: If a vacancy occurs, will the person's share of the costs increase? _____

Senior Adult Condominiums

If you're considering a senior adult condominium, ask the building manager the following questions. (The first three questions only apply if the condominium is still being constructed.) Note: Before you speak with the building manager, you may want to talk to the owner of the unit first to see if an acceptable price can be negotiated. Don't waste precious time investigating the facility if the elderly person cannot afford it or no unit is available.

When will the unit be ready to occupy? _____

How much say does the elderly person have in selecting fixtures, wall coverings? _____

_____

How many units have actually been sold (excluding those for which only deposits have been made)?

_____

May we have a copy of the condominium documents? (Have a lawyer review the documents.) _____

May we have a copy of the condominium association's rules and regulations? (Have a lawyer review the documents.) _____

Is there any litigation pending? _____

Is the present owner current on all fees and charges? If not, who is responsible for paying them? _____

What restrictions exist on the sale of the unit? _____

_____

Does the condominium association have to approve new owners?

_____

Who's responsible for maintenance? _____

Who's responsible for security? _____

What are the maintenance fees? _____

When did they last increase? _____

When are maintenance fees scheduled to increase again? _____

Are any changes planned to the common areas?

_____

Will these changes increase fees and expenses? _____

Who is in charge of the owner's association?_____

When are taxes due? How are they assessed?_____

_____

Is there a list of approved home healthcare aides available?

_____

Is transportation provided for shopping, doctor visits, and so on?

_____

Are there any assisted-living facilities nearby?

_____

Rental Units

The following questions apply to senior apartments, senior retirement centers, retirement hotels, Section 202 housing, subsidized congregate housing, public housing, and supported housing for seniors with disabilities. Again, make sure that the elderly person can afford the unit and can meet any eligibility requirements before you investigate the facility.

Is the unit ready for occupancy? _____

Is the unit delivered "as is" (same paint, carpet, appliances, and so on)?

_____

Is the unit's current condition documented in writing?_____

Does the renter have a say in refurbishment before moving in?

_____

Who's responsible for maintenance? _____

Can the renter bring in furniture and other personal possessions?

_____

Do personal possessions remain the property of the renter? _____

Are there restrictions on guests or visitors?

_____

How much turnover has there been in the last six months?

_____

Is subleasing permitted? _____

Are there restrictions on someone else moving in with the elderly person?

_____

_____

May we have a copy of the rules and regulations? _____

Is there any litigation pending? _____

Are you planning any changes that could increase the monthly fees and expenses? _____

_____

Can residents control their own heating and air conditioning? _____

Does the building have a sprinkler system in case of fire?_____

Does each unit have working smoke detectors? _____

Do residents practice fire drills? _____

What is the smoking policy? _____

Is the building secured during the day? In the evening?_____

Is transportation available? _____

Are there any organized social events? _____

Is there a tenant's organization? If so, who's in charge of it?

_____

How are problems among residents handled? _____

Who pays for utilities? _____

Is there an extra fee to connect to cable TV? _____

How much notice is required before moving out? _____

What about in an emergency, such as a transfer to a hospital or nursing home, or the loss of ADLs (see page 76)? _____

_____

What happens if the elderly person no longer meets the eligibility requirements? _____

_____

Under what circumstances can the lease be broken? _____

_____

Continuing Care Retirement Communities (CCRCs) and Life Care Communities

These questions address issues that are specific to CCRCs and life care communities. You may find that the questions in the previous sections are relevant here as well, especially those for rental units.

What are the entrance and monthly fees? Are future increases capped?

_____

What services are included in the fees? _____

What services are not included in the fees?_____

Will future expansion plans or growing healthcare costs affect the monthly fee? _____

_____

Is any portion of the entrance fee refundable? _____

What happens if the elderly person remarries? _____

What if the new spouse is another resident? What if he or she is not?

_____

If a married couple is admitted, what happens if one spouse dies?

_____

What fees must continue to be paid if the resident moves to an assisted-living facility or a nursing home? _____

_____

Who determines the elderly person's level of care and housing?

_____

Is the facility accredited by the Continuing Care Accreditation Commission? _____

Are the assisted-living facility and nursing home licensed by the state?

_____

Is the nursing home certified for participation in Medicare and Medicaid? _____

May we have copies of the ownership and financial information? (Have a lawyer review the documents.) _____

Under what circumstances might a resident be required to leave?

_____

When a resident is transferred to the assisted-living facility or nursing home, do the fees increase? How soon? _____

Are there special facilities on the premises—doctors, therapists, bank, pharmacy, convenience store? _____

_____

Can home care services be provided in the apartment unit? _____

Are special dietary requirements taken into account? _____

Can a requirement to move to a higher level of care be appealed?

_____

If the resident moves out, how much time is allowed for the removal of personal possessions? _____

Shared Housing

"Shared housing" refers to small group housing, adult foster care, matched housing, and Eldercare Housing Opportunity (ECHO). Most of the questions that follow apply to all of these options except ECHO. (ECHO is mainly a cost and zoning-law issue.)

Remember, adult foster care and matched housing both involve one-on-one relationships between the elderly person and a caregiver. The selection process involves checking references, working out the terms of the live-in arrangement, and assessing compatibility during the interview. (Compatibility and expectations are important issues in shared housing. Read Moving In with the Caregiver beginning on page 127 for a discussion of these issues.)

How many people are allowed to live here?_____

How many people live here right now? _____

What services are included in the basic charge?_____

What services would the elderly person have to pay for separately?

_____

Does the basic charge increase if a vacancy occurs? _____

May we have a copy of the admission agreement and any rules or regulations? _____

Who is in charge of enforcing the rules? _____

Under what circumstances can a resident be forced to leave?

_____

Does the resident have to give notice if he or she leaves voluntarily?

_____

May we see the private room(s) the elderly person would occupy?

_____

Are there any restrictions on bringing in the resident's own furniture, television, telephone, and so on?_____

What services or tasks are residents supposed to perform? How often?

_____

What happens if they cannot or will not perform these tasks?

_____

How to Find Residential Housing

What You Need to Know

When it becomes clear that the elderly person needs custodial or nursing care outside the home, the housing selection process changes considerably. It is much more difficult to select residential housing than independent housing, since direct care to the elderly person is usually involved.

For one thing, the elderly person is less likely to be involved in the decision, which places most of the burden on the caregiver and family. Also, while a move to congregate housing, a senior apartment, a shared living facility, and many assisted-living facilities can be approached in positive terms—for example, as a way to maintain the person's independence despite his or her declining abilities—a move to a residential care building cannot be explained away. If the elderly person is unaware of his or her surroundings because of illness, accident, or disease, this may not be much of an issue. Nevertheless, the caregiver and family may feel a mixture of guilt, helplessness, and concern about whether or not they have made the right decision, especially if the elderly person opposed the move or had hoped to move in with a family member.

Prepare for the Unexpected

If you believe that residential housing will be needed sometime in the future, look for that facility now, before the need arises. High-quality residential care facilities—whether assisted-living environments or nursing homes—usually have long waiting lists. Finding the best facility and getting on its waiting list is a prudent decision, even if it requires a deposit. (Be sure the deposit can be refunded if the admission never takes place or if a room isn't available when it is needed.) Also, it doesn't hurt to look at facilities with different levels of care. An assisted-living facility or personal care home may look like the logical choice today, but if the elderly person has a stroke or accident tomorrow, a nursing home would be more appropriate. Try to find the best facility for each level of care.

Although many elderly people move to a residential care facility because their condition has changed, some are admitted when their caregivers can no longer meet their responsibilities. Caring for another person, especially one who requires twenty-four-hour nursing care, is a serious commitment. Caregivers may run into a host of personal difficulties, such as illness or financial problems. Or, the family may realize that their efforts to keep the elderly person out of a nursing home are chiefly for their own benefit and no longer in the person's best interest. Plan for the unexpected. Select a residential facility before any of these situations occur.

Financial Planning

In addition to selecting a facility for the future, take advantage of the opportunity to make financial plans as well. Depending on the location, type, quality, and level of services provided, the cost of a residential facility can run from $15,000 to over $100,000 a year.

Unless the elderly person qualifies for third-party payment (payment by insurance, Medicare, Medicaid, and so forth), residential care must be privately funded by the elderly person or his or her family. If the elderly person will be admitted to a residential facility, and you think he or she may be eligible for Medicare, Medicaid, long-term care insurance, or health insurance, be absolutely certain of the coverage and its expected duration before you make a commitment. Remember, too, that there are often limits to third-party payments. The shortfall—the difference between the monthly bill and what insurance or another third party will pay—will be the elderly person's responsibility.

Both the *Vital Information Form* (pages 9–33) and *Financial Worksheets* (pages 39–54) have sections to help caregivers and financial planners prepare for the cost of future residential and medical care. Paying for Nursing Homes, which begins on page 148, includes a general explanation of payment options specifically for nursing home care. Because this is a technical and ever-evolving area that differs from state to state, a detailed explanation of each option would be incomplete at best. Other books and resources offer advice and counseling in this area, but specific questions should be directed to a financial planner or an estate or elderlaw attorney.

Before You Begin …

With any residential housing, you will face two questions—how to choose a residential care facility, and how to know if you've made the right choice. No matter what alternative you select, your decision can and should be reviewed later, particularly if it was made during a crisis or if the elderly person's needs change. Beyond that, there are two ways you can help to ensure your decision will be in the best interest of the elderly person.

1. Involve the family. Choosing a residential care facility is a difficult decision, and it's important to involve other family members every step of the way. If a family member has not yet accepted the fact that the elderly person needs residential care, he or she is unlikely to approve of any of the facilities you choose. Furthermore, if family members haven't helped narrow down the choices, their expectations, observations, and opinions may be totally unrealistic.

Try to get as many people involved in the decision as possible. This way, important concerns about a facility are more likely to surface, and your chances of reaching a consensus improve.

Ideally, the elderly person will visit the facilities under consideration. In reality, however, he or she

may refuse to go, act uncooperatively, or have no frame of reference on which to base a decision. Even if the person acknowledges the necessity of the move, the options available may seem unacceptable to him or her. Remember, it's the elderly person's life. Unless there's a real question about mental competency, the person should help decide where he or she is going to live.

2. Consider the future. When selecting a facility, consider both immediate and long-term needs. (You can sort out financial resources and weigh quality of care later.) If the elderly person needs physical or IV therapy, the facility must be able to provide these services. If the person has a mental disability, such as severe dementia, the facility must provide the staff, equipment, and physical surroundings necessary to care for this condition.

If you know that the move will be permanent, try to anticipate how the person's condition will progress. Talk to a doctor, geriatric care manager, therapist, social worker, or home healthcare agency, and make sure you understand the elderly person's prognosis. Use this information to determine if a prospective facility will be able to handle the elderly person's needs in the future. An assisted-living facility may seem appropriate in the short-term, but if the person's condition is likely to deteriorate quickly, and you know that nursing care will eventually be required, you have two options: (1) look for a facility that provides a higher level of care than is currently necessary (such as a nursing home), or (2) choose an assisted-living facility now and continue to investigate nursing homes for the future.

It's important to remember, however, that unless the elderly person needs skilled nursing care, you should not admit him or her to a nursing home as a private pay resident. If you do and his or her funds run out, Medicaid will not cover the elderly person's care. (Medicaid will only pay for skilled nursing care.) The nursing home will discharge the elderly person, and he or she will not have the funds to pay for an assisted-living facility.

How to Find the Right Facility

Unless you're familiar with the residential care resources in your community, you will want to seek recommendations. Start with the elderly person's doctor. The doctor can tell you what level of care is needed and for how long. The doctor can also help you choose the most appropriate type of housing and explain if special facilities, services, or therapies are likely to be required. Finally, the doctor may recommend that you consider or avoid certain facilities. It is important to remember that a doctor should not be asked to make the decision for you, but his or her opinion should be given a lot of weight, especially if the doctor has experience with the facilities you are considering.

If the elderly person is moving from a hospital to a residential care facility, ask the hospital discharge planner for recommendations. Be aware, however, that the discharge planner's job is to get people out of the hospital as quickly as possible—he or she may recommend a home that is certain to take the patient.

If the elderly person has special needs or problems, such as Alzheimer's disease, national associations and local support groups can direct you toward good programs or facilities in your community. (See chapter 7 for a list of these organizations.)

The state ombudsman's office is a free resource that can help you sort out nursing home options. (To contact the office in your state, see chapter 7.) This office investigates complaints and acts as an advocate for residents, so staff members are familiar with the quality of care provided by long-term care facilities in your area. While they're not allowed to make specific recommendations, you can learn about the quality of certain facilities by asking about survey results and the frequency of complaints. This

office can also direct you to other resources in your local community.

Clergy, geriatric care managers, home healthcare workers, other caregivers, your local Area Agency on Aging, and the elderly person's friends may also have recommendations. The more time you have, the more networking you can do. In a small community, a lot of networking may not be necessary because of the limited number of facilities available. However, the comments you hear may reveal potential problems or issues you should discuss during your visits to these facilities.

Special Considerations

1. Location. If the elderly person lives far away, you might consider moving him or her to a facility that is closer to the caregiver. The decision will depend on specific considerations: Can the person be safely moved? Do facilities in both locations meet his or her needs? Does the person want to move? How do other family members feel?

If the elderly person is moving to a nursing home, there may be third-party payment considerations as well. For example, if he or she would be moving to a different state, does that state's Medicaid program have a minimum residency requirement before benefits are payable? If the person must change Medigap providers, could there be problems with waiting periods or preexisting conditions?

If the elderly person no longer has ties to his or her community, it may be best to move to a new location where there will be more visitors. However, even under the best circumstances, a move to a residential facility is traumatic and disorienting for everyone involved. If the real motive for the move is the caregiver's convenience, and the elderly person would be leaving behind his or her community and friends, the caregiver may not be acting in the elderly person's best interest.

2. Visitors. Try to choose a facility that's convenient to visitors. Regular visits by family, friends, clergy, doctors, and others are vital to the elderly person's quality of life. Naturally, if he or she requires a facility with special services, this will take precedence.

3. Religious and cultural preferences. Sometimes elderly people have strong religious, ethnic, or cultural preferences that will override geographical convenience. The elderly person may have a strong preference for a Catholic or Jewish nursing home, for example, or a facility where the staff speaks Spanish. It is disorienting enough to be uprooted from your home and friends. To also be ripped from your culture may create severe psychological and emotional problems that will make adjustment virtually impossible.

4. Surveys and inspection reports. If the elderly person is moving to a nursing home, be sure to look at recent state or federal surveys of the facilities you are considering. A review of the facility's operation by a team of inspectors, a survey attempts to measure the quality of life in the facility and the care being provided. You can order the last three surveys from the HCFA (Health Care Financing Administration), which oversees Medicare and Medicaid programs. Your ombudsman (see chapter 7) can also tell you how to order this "Oscar" report and how much it will cost. You will need the facility's name and Medicare provider number.

Survey reports are difficult to understand, and it's often impossible for a layperson to distinguish a serious violation from a technical one. If the facility is still licensed and certified for participation in Medicare or Medicaid, you know that the inspectors ultimately decided that minimal standards of care were being met. Don't assume that many deficiencies indicate a bad facility, or that few deficiencies indicate a good one. Surveys do not recognize excellent care; they simply identify problems to assure that minimum standards of care are being

met. It's also important to note that an old survey is no indication of the facility's current quality, regardless of its content. Residential care facilities, especially nursing homes, generally have high employee turnover at all levels, and the quality of care can change overnight.

While it's important to review surveys, you shouldn't give them too much weight unless the results vary dramatically from your observations. Generally, your observations will confirm the overall survey results. Higher-quality facilities will usually have better surveys, and marginal facilities will have more deficiencies.

The most recent survey results should be posted in the facility or otherwise available for review. (If you are told that they have been lost or stolen, this is a red flag and you should definitely talk to the ombudsman.) Surveys take several days to complete and usually occur every nine to fifteen months. If the facility has violated any regulations, these deficiencies are noted in a report. The facility must respond to each deficiency by filing a plan of correction. A deficiency may be a technical noncompliance, or it may be a serious violation involving a loss of licensure or loss of Medicare or Medicaid certification. Depending on the nature and severity of the violations, a follow-up inspection may be required. The facility has the right to appeal a deficiency and contest any citation or civil penalty. This process can take months, and the results are seldom published at the facility, regardless of the outcome.

5. Restraint policy. By law, all nursing homes are required to have a restraint reduction program. Either the director of nursing or the administrator of the nursing home should be able to discuss this program with you. The law says that physical and chemical restraints may only be used to treat medical conditions or to ensure the safety of residents. You should note, however, that a blanket "no restraints" policy can be as shortsighted as an over-aggressive use of restraints. Ask about the facility's policy on the use of restraints and find out how they monitor compliance with that policy.

It is equally important to observe the nursing home's residents. Are a substantial number of them wearing wheelchair belts that they can't remove, or are they restrained by geri-chairs, hard mitts, or bed alarms? While some restraints are appropriate for safety reasons, excessive use of restraints may mean that the facility is understaffed.

6. Residents' bill of rights. By law, every nursing home must post a residents' bill of rights, although many residents are too sick, disoriented, or mentally ill to understand it. During your visit, it's worth a few minutes of your time to read the residents' bill of rights. Find out how the facility informs residents and families of their rights and how it ensures that these rights are protected.

7. Family council. Lastly, in addition to the legally mandated resident council, many nursing homes also have a family council. The family council is an excellent source of information, especially about potential problems and difficult staff members. If it meets regularly, it may be your best resource. Expect the members to be interested, caring family members who advocate for the residents. Their views of the management, staff, and quality of life and care at the facility are a good indicator of the real state of affairs.

Touring Facilities

Once you've narrowed down your list to two or three places, try to visit each facility twice—once during the day and again around dinnertime, on a weekend, or first thing in the morning. During the first visit, you'll get a formal tour and meet with the people in charge to ask your list of questions. On the second visit, try to get a feel for the facility when it's busy and perhaps short-staffed. On this visit, what you observe is more important than what you are told.

If you're not familiar with residential care facilities, remember that they are not acute care hospitals. Generally, people are not in bed or even in their rooms. They are wandering the halls, sitting in wheelchairs, socializing, getting a bath, eating, or visiting with family or friends. There is always some degree of chaos, and residents wander around in various stages of dress. It is a loud environment; poor hearing leads to loud conversations among residents and staff.

During your second visit, take the time to ask the staff, residents, and the residents' families about the facility's services and care. Watch how staff members address the residents, how alert and well-groomed the residents are, and how aware the residents' families are about what is going on there. All of this will help you get a feel for the facility, which will play an important role in your decision.

When you visit a facility, bring along one of the residential care forms (page 152 or 155). The first form is from the Health Care Financing Administration's *Guide to Choosing a Nursing Home*, although most of the questions are just as applicable to assisted-living facilities. It's designed to capture your impressions rather than answer specific questions, and it will provide a basis for comparing facilities. The second form contains questions that cover a range of issues. Because it is long, you may wish to focus on only those questions that concern you. If you need help interpreting any of the answers, you should talk to a geriatric care manager, discharge planner, or elderlaw attorney.

Once you've seen the residential care facilities, the best choice will probably be self-evident. Typically, several factors will combine to tip the balance in favor of one facility. If the best alternative does not stand out, however, it's time to return to the beginning—balancing the elderly person's needs, his or her finances, and community resources. With a better understanding of each area, the caregiver will know which should be given the most weight.

Admission: Knowing If You've Made the Right Choice

When you choose a residential care facility, you strive to make the best decision based on the information available. However, the only way to know if you've made the right decision is to watch and wait. Once the elderly person has been admitted, you must continually monitor the quality of care, the quality of life, and whether the facility and staff are performing as expected. Keep in mind the following:

• Don't be too quick to judge. This kind of transition is seldom easy for the elderly or their caregivers. Some people need time to adjust their expectations about a residential care facility. Also, the stress of the change may cause the elderly person's condition to deteriorate at first, but it should improve within a few days or weeks.

• If you think there's a problem, make sure you have all the facts before you take any sudden action. Rumors start and change in the telling and retelling, and someone with an ax to grind may try to create problems.

• Once you're part of the system, you can look within it for help and guidance. Talking to the ombudsman, other families, family council members, and the administrator can help put a situation in perspective. Ironically, the more technical a matter, the easier it may be to find someone to explain it. In many situations, the bigger the issue, the easier it may be to find a solution because of the number of people affected.

Quality of Life

The most difficult problems to resolve usually involve quality of life. These problems tend to involve personality disputes between residents, and sometimes between residents and staff. The elderly may not get along with a roommate, they may think they're being abused by another resident, or they may not feel accepted by the community. Perhaps they have few friends. They might keep to themselves and refuse to participate in activities or go to the dining room or lounge. Depending on the severity of the problem, the elderly person's condition, and your ability to correct the underlying issues, a move to a different facility may be required.

Sometimes, undiagnosed depression or a change in medication could cause the elderly person to have problems adjusting; they could even create a change in his or her personality. Before moving the elderly person to a new facility, talk to a doctor about the possibility of depression, and discuss the side effects of any medications the person is taking and how they might interact with other medicines.

Quality of Care

Quality of care issues tend to reflect problems with the staff. If the elderly person is dirty or unkempt; is not being fully dressed and groomed; is being physically or chemically restrained; has unexplained skin tears, bruises, or bed sores; complains about particular staff people; or refuses to discuss the staff out of fear or intimidation, the problem needs to be addressed swiftly, especially if it appears to affect only the elderly person. If staff members appear evasive or cannot provide acceptable answers to your concerns, don't hesitate to raise the issue with the administrator, director of nursing, or ombudsman.

If you're concerned about the quality of care, you may need to ask the elderly person specific questions, such as the following:

• What did you eat today?
• How much water did you drink?
• Who gave you a bath?
• Did you move your bowels?
• Did you urinate? How much?
• Did you take your medications?
• Are you in pain? Where does it hurt?

Questions like "How are you? How do you feel today?" won't be very helpful. Specific questions, on the other hand, force the elderly person to discuss the care being provided. You may have to ask a staff member about these issues if the elderly person is unable to answer.

When confronted with quality of life or quality of care issues, record your thoughts, observations, and any other relevant information in a daily diary to document what is said and done. Keeping a detailed record and getting specific answers to your questions is the only way to document a problem.

Regular, random visits keep staff members on their toes. If you cannot visit regularly, ask someone you trust to look in on the elderly person and report back to you. If you have a question or problem or feel dissatisfied with the care, confront the issue as soon as possible.

Getting to Know the Staff

Although staff members generally have a high level of turnover, it's important to get to know the nurses and aides who work with the elderly person, especially on night and weekend shifts. They are the primary caregivers now. Even though they're almost always underpaid and overworked, these caregivers determine the quality of care the elderly person receives. If they can see that you care because you visit regularly and are holding them to a high (but not impossible) standard, they will provide a higher level of care. Getting to know them and recognizing their efforts with kindness and an occasional gift or thank-you note will also help ensure high-quality care.

The reverse is also true. If you don't visit, are ignorant about what is going on in the facility, are rude toward the staff, make frivolous complaints about the care (especially to supervisors or to the ombudsman), fail to appreciate staff members' other duties, or generally become a pain to have around, it will likely have a negative effect on the

quality of care. Nurse aides have a difficult job. While you should certainly expect professionalism, it's critical to appreciate their hard work and the difficulties they encounter.

Occasionally, racial or ethnic differences between residents, their families, and staff members may cause problems. If such a situation arises, try to be diplomatic. If the problem persists and is not corrected, don't hesitate to speak to the administrator, director of nursing, or ombudsman. If necessary, file a complaint with the state.

When to Move to a Different Facility

The trauma of moving to a residential facility is difficult enough, and a decision to move the resident to a new facility should not be made hastily. You may be better off directing your efforts toward identifying and correcting problems at the current facility.

Aside from the facility closing, there are only three reasons to seriously consider moving the resident to another facility:

1. The person's physical, mental, or emotional condition has changed, and the facility can no longer meet his or her needs. If this occurs, discuss it with the elderly person, his or her doctor, and the staff. If a change is necessary, you'll have to begin the selection process all over again.

2. There are serious quality of life or quality of care issues that don't improve, despite your attempts to resolve them through the staff, the family council, the administrator, and even the state. If the problem only seems to affect one person, ask yourself if your expectations are realistic before you make a decision. Of course, even if the problem is isolated—or if the elderly person is causing his or her own problems—it may still be necessary to move to a different facility.

3. The facility evicts the elderly person for nonpayment or for breaking the rules. State laws and regulations make eviction an extraordinary remedy, but hundreds, if not thousands, of nursing home residents are evicted every year, usually for nonpayment. Occasionally, Medicaid will refuse to pay for care if the elderly person fails to qualify (as in the case of a large asset being transferred just before the person applied for Medicaid.)

Paying for Nursing Homes

There are several ways to pay for nursing home care: through Medicare, Medicaid, private funds, long-term care insurance, a managed care arrangement (through the elderly person's private health insurance), or a combination of these. Even with the help of Medicaid or insurance, there's a good chance that the elderly person—or his or her caregiver—will be responsible for at least part of the nursing home payments. However, if families plan far enough ahead of time, elderlaw attorneys and financial planners can work with the elderly person to create a plan that minimizes his or her share of nursing home costs. (See page 149 for more information on Medicaid planning.) A common misconception is that this sort of planning will reduce an elderly person's share of assisted-living costs, as well. It will not, since Medicaid generally does not pay for care in assisted-living facilities.

The following is an introduction to the various ways you can pay for nursing home care. For additional information, your local Area Agency on Aging and many of the organizations and hotlines listed in chapter 7 provide information on different payment alternatives. Also, publications from federal and state agencies that administer Medicare and Medicaid explain these programs in detail. In addition, insurance companies, insurance and financial consultants, and consumer groups have written extensively about long-term care insurance. Health insurers, financial consultants, and elderlaw attorneys can discuss how managed care options operate and what a patient's rights are.

The list that follows is not comprehensive, and you will need to seek professional advice about paying for any form of residential housing, including nursing homes. When you meet with a professional, be sure to bring the completed *Vital Information Form* (pages 9–33) and *Financial Worksheets* (pages 39–54), as well as copies of any applicable healthcare or long-term care insurance policies.

Medicare

With few (and limited) exceptions, Medicare will not pay for care in an assisted-living facility or nursing home, nor will it cover chronic conditions. Medicare is an insurance program. It will cover acute medical care, home healthcare, hospitalization, prescriptions, and therapy, but it has narrow limits for long-term care coverage. It will only pay if sub-acute or highly skilled nursing services are required (certain Medicare Part B services may also be covered). Where Medicare does cover nursing home care, the nursing home must be Medicare-certified.

There is a 100-day lifetime limit for skilled nursing care. If Medicare will cover the nursing home care, it will pay for the first twenty days without requiring a deductible payment. The deductible amount changes every year.

Many nursing homes are not Medicare-certified. Those that are will usually take a potential Medicare patient if they can provide the level of care that the patient needs. If the elderly person is in the hospital awaiting admission to a nursing home, and the doctor, discharge planner, or nursing home admissions coordinator tells you that the elderly person might be eligible for Medicare, you should apply immediately. If Medicare pays, the elderly person would only be responsible for the deductible and for expenses not covered by Medicare, such as laundry or beautician services. Some of these expenses might be picked up by Medicare Supplemental Insurance (Medigap).

Medicaid

Medicaid (Medi-Cal, in California) is a federal/state entitlement program for the poor. As an entitlement program, Medicaid only makes payments if the elderly person meets certain qualifications. The rules vary from state to state. Each state program differs in eligibility requirements, how and when services are provided, the amount paid, the elderly person's ability to choose a provider, and how the quality of care is assessed. If the elderly person meets all the eligibility requirements, Medicaid will begin payment after he or she applies for benefits. If the person doesn't meet all the requirements, benefits won't begin until assets have been "spent down" to the point that the elderly person becomes poor, as defined by Medicaid.

Once Medicaid begins to pay for long-term care, the elderly person may or may not be required to share part of the cost, depending on his or her level of income. When there is a "share of cost" payment, it usually isn't very much.

The process of applying for Medicaid usually begins after admission to a long-term care facility. Again, state requirements vary. If any of the elderly person's assets have been transferred within five years of his or her admission to the facility, you should not apply for Medicaid until you speak with a professional who understands Medicaid reimbursement. He or she will probably want to see the *Vital Information Form* (beginning on page 9) and *Financial Worksheets* (beginning on page 39), because the elderly person's assets, income, and asset transfers will affect eligibility.

Medicaid often reimburses facilities for less than what the nursing care and other services really cost. Therefore, most facilities "cost shift"—that is, they rely on private payers, insurance, and even Medicare to make up the difference. For this reason, most facilities don't want more Medicaid residents than they already have. Discriminating against Medicaid residents is against the law in most states; nevertheless, many facilities do it by limiting the number of Medicaid beds available. If the elderly person will be a Medicaid admission, assume that his or her choice of facilities will be limited, especially if he or she needs special care, such as an Alzheimer's unit.

The importance of Medicaid planning cannot be overemphasized. If the elderly person doesn't plan ahead, his or her assets most likely will be used to pay for nursing home care until these assets are exhausted. However, only a qualified professional can assure that Medicaid planning will have the intended result. Medicaid planning does not mean "transfer everything now"; it usually involves saving some assets and transferring others. There are technical rules about the following:

• Which assets count in determining net worth, and which do not

• Which assets are "deemed" to be owned by the elderly person

• Whether there is asset recovery after death (where the state recoups some of its Medicaid payments from the estate)

• How Medicaid treats the "community spouse" (when one spouse is admitted to a nursing home, the one at home is referred to as a "community spouse")

• How the "lookback period" changes for asset transfers (generally, a period of up to five years before an application for Medicaid is filed will be reviewed for asset transfers from the Medicaid applicant)

• How Medicaid treats monthly income to determine the elderly person's "share of cost"

It is worth noting here that Medicaid planning is a two-way street: Just as planning can be done to minimize the use of private resources for long-term care, planning can also be done to ensure that enough private resources are available to assure admittance into the facility of choice. Ask your Medicaid financial planner about the Rule of Halves.

Private Pay

Many people enter residential care facilities as private pay residents, but few maintain this status, especially if they require nursing care for a long period of time. Private pay rates average between $1,200 and $3,000 a month in an assisted-living facility, and between $3,500 and $9,000 a month in a nursing home. Although the cost is high, it is not exorbitant, especially when compared to the cost of providing the same level of care in the home (with twenty-four-hour nursing, home healthcare, and housekeeping services) or in an acute care hospital (at $800 to over $1,000 a day). Nevertheless, it's a substantial amount to pay, and the cost of long-term residential care is likely to wipe out the elderly person's savings over time. Most providers are sensitive to this and may negotiate payment terms.

While it's against the law to require a deposit from a resident admitted under Medicare or Medicaid, it's generally not against the law to require one of a private pay resident. Without a deposit, the facility could lose too much money if the elderly person doesn't pay. With Medicare and Medicaid, the risk to the facility is far lower, since the payer is the federal or state government. Sometimes, if the elderly person's resources are limited, the caregiver or other family members can sign a contract agreeing to pay for so many months or years of care. (In most states, you cannot sign this agreement unless you have access to the elderly person's funds.) The contract can be drafted to limit the family's financial exposure and help the person gain admission to a facility that will not take a Medicaid patient.

While the elderly person's payment status shouldn't affect his or her quality of care, it may affect the quality of facility available. Unless a facility is full or space for the appropriate gender is not available, private pay residents will generally be admitted to any facility they choose.

Because consumer protection legislation makes issues of nonpayment harder to resolve, facilities are more aggressive now about evicting residents who routinely do not pay on time. Additionally, many facilities pursue legal recourse against anyone intentionally involved in fraud, such as a son listed as an authorized signer on an elderly person's checking account who removes funds so that there's no money to pay the facility.

Long-Term Care Insurance

"Long-term care insurance" refers to a source of funds belonging to a private pay resident in a residential care facility. In a way, it's a savings account dedicated to paying for residential care. Long-term care insurance is becoming increasingly accepted as a way to preserve assets in old age. Although it has been around for a number of years, long-term care insurance was initially plagued by consumer complaints. Many people paid for policies but were unable to collect the benefits because of overly restrictive provisions about when the benefits would be paid. In recent years, consumer protection and industry competition have combined to create a range of acceptable policies that can be tailored to individual needs. Policies are relatively inexpensive, especially if they are acquired when the insured person is under the age of fifty.

In most cases, the policies provide a set daily payment when certain conditions arise, such as the inability to perform two or more Activities of Daily Living (see page 76). The payments are made to the elderly person and can be used to pay long-term care providers. Some national nursing home chains are starting to write contracts in which they agree to accept payment from a long-term care insurance company as payment in full. For now, however, it is still "buyer beware."

Chapter 7 lists some resources to check before acquiring a policy.

If the elderly person has long-term care insurance and is about to be admitted to a long-term care facility, be absolutely certain that any preconditions for payment are satisfied to the letter. For example, in many policies, patients must have a hospital stay before they are admitted to a nursing home. Otherwise, insurance won't pay for the nursing home. If you have any questions, contact the insurance agent or an elderlaw attorney before admitting the elderly person to a long-term care facility. Also, let prospective facilities know that long-term care insurance is involved. If they have experience with the carrier, they may know if there are any hidden pitfalls to avoid.

Managed Care Providers

Managed care organizations, or health maintenance organizations (HMOs), mainly cover short-term acute care in hospitals and various outpatient settings. However, more and more HMOs are beginning to pay for residential care services. Some will contract with nursing homes to provide services on a case-by-case basis. (These nursing homes will generally provide sub-acute care for patients released from a hospital until they are well enough to return home.) The role that HMOs play in paying for residential care is likely to increase as Medicare and Medicaid permit—or force—beneficiaries to have services provided and paid for by managed care providers instead of the government. New York, for example, is in the process of moving all of its Medicaid beneficiaries into managed care programs.

Managed care providers must designate or approve a residential care facility before they will pay for an elderly person's care. The provider will generally contract with a specific long-term care facility, although the elderly person can often choose from a group of approved facilities.

Medicare and Medicaid measure quality of care by reviewing facilities as a whole against a set of regulations. Managed care providers, on the other hand, tend to measure quality by comparing individual cases to the expected outcomes.

HCFA NURSING HOME CHECKLIST

This checklist, developed by the Health Care Financing Administration, is designed to help you evaluate and compare nursing homes. It's a good idea to make several copies of this checklist so that you will have a new one for each home you visit.

PART 1—BASIC INFORMATION

Name of Nursing Home: _____

Address: _____

_____

Phone: _____

Cultural/Religious Affiliation (if any): _____

Medicaid Certified?	yes	no
Medicare Certified?	yes	no
Admitting New Residents?	yes	no
Convenient Location?	yes	no
Is home capable of meeting your special care needs?	yes	no

For parts two through five, rate the nursing home on a scale from one to ten, with ten being a perfect score.

PART 2—QUALITY OF LIFE

1. Are residents treated respectfully by staff at all times?   1 2 3 4 5 6 7 8 9 10

2. Are residents dressed appropriately and well-groomed?   1 2 3 4 5 6 7 8 9 10

3. Does staff make an effort to meet the needs of each resident?   1 2 3 4 5 6 7 8 9 10

4. Is there a variety of activities to meet the needs
   of individual residents?   1 2 3 4 5 6 7 8 9 10

5. Is the food attractive and tasty? (sample a meal if possible)   1 2 3 4 5 6 7 8 9 10

6. Are resident rooms decorated with personal articles?   1 2 3 4 5 6 7 8 9 10

7. Is the environment homelike?   1 2 3 4 5 6 7 8 9 10

8. Do common areas and resident rooms contain comfortable furniture?   1 2 3 4 5 6 7 8 9 10

9. Does the facility have a family and resident's council?   1 2 3 4 5 6 7 8 9 10

10. Does the facility have contact with outside groups of volunteers?   1 2 3 4 5 6 7 8 9 10

PART 3—QUALITY OF CARE

11. Does staff encourage residents to act independently?   1 2 3 4 5 6 7 8 9 10

12. Does facility staff respond quickly to calls for assistance?   1 2 3 4 5 6 7 8 9 10

13. Are residents and family involved in resident care planning?   1 2 3 4 5 6 7 8 9 10

14. Does the home offer appropriate therapies (physical, speech, etc.)?   1 2 3 4 5 6 7 8 9 10

15. Does the nursing home have an arrangement with a nearby hospital?   1 2 3 4 5 6 7 8 9 10

PART 4—SAFETY

16. Are there enough staff to appropriately provide care to residents?   1 2 3 4 5 6 7 8 9 10

17. Are there handrails in the hallways and grab bars in bathrooms?   1 2 3 4 5 6 7 8 9 10

18. Is the inside of the home in good repair and are exits clearly marked? 1 2 3 4 5 6 7 8 9 10

19. Are spills and other accidents cleaned up quickly?   1 2 3 4 5 6 7 8 9 10

20. Are the hallways free of clutter and well-lighted?   1 2 3 4 5 6 7 8 9 10

PART 5—OTHER CONCERNS

21. Does the home have outdoor areas (patios, etc.) for resident use?   1 2 3 4 5 6 7 8 9 10

22. Does the home provide an updated list of references?   1 2 3 4 5 6 7 8 9 10

23. Are the latest survey reports and list of resident rights posted?   1 2 3 4 5 6 7 8 9 10

24. (Your Concern)

_____

_____

_____

25. (Your Concern)

_____

_____

_____

26. Additional Comments

_____

_____

_____

_____

_____

_____

_____

_____

This checklist may be reproduced and circulated. It is designed to be used in concert with the Health Care Financing Administration's booklet, *The Guide to Choosing a Nursing Home*. This booklet can be obtained by calling (800) 638-6833.

RESIDENTIAL HOUSING FORM

The following questions get to the heart of a long-term care facility. They will help give you a feel for the facility, its staff, its resources, its philosophy of care, and its flexibility in meeting the elderly person's changing needs.

If you will be reviewing these questions yourself, without the help of a consultant or professional, you may want to stick to the starred questions. While all these questions provide relevant information to someone who understands the residential care industry, average caregivers should focus on those that are most important to them and trust their observations. Tailor your questions to the issues you are most concerned about.

A different form should be completed for each facility visited. This form may be used in conjunction with the *HCFA Nursing Home Checklist* (beginning on page 152).

Basic Information

*Facility name_____

*Address _____

*Telephone number_____ *Fax number_____

*Administrator_____ *How long there? _____

*Director of nursing (if applicable)_____ *How long there? _____

Other key staff (if applicable)_____

Assistant administrator _____

Assistant director of nursing _____

Quality assurance nurse _____

*Business office manager _____

Director of social services _____

Activities director _____

*Admissions coordinator _____

*Facility license number _____

*Licensed by which state agency? _____

*How many beds are in the facility?_____ *How many of the beds are occupied?_____

*Is the facility accredited by the Joint Commission on Accreditation of Healthcare Organizations (JCAHO)?_____ When was the most recent survey? _____

Is the facility organized as a for-profit or not-for-profit? _____

Has ownership changed within the last five years? _____

A Family Caregiver's Guide to Planning and Decision Making for the Elderly © 1999 James A. Wilkinson

Is the facility part of a chain of affiliated or related facilities? _____

Are there any affiliated or related facilities in the local community?_____

*Is there a medical director?_____ Who is the medical director? _____

How can the medical director be contacted? _____

*How often is the medical director usually in the facility? _____

Is the medical director on call twenty-four-hours a day? _____

*Will the elderly person's doctor be able to provide services here? _____

Is that doctor caring for any residents in the facility at the moment? _____

Will the doctor need the facility's permission to visit the patient? _____

If the resident's doctor can't be contacted promptly, when does the facility's medical director become involved?_____

What if there is a dispute between the doctor and the medical director over treatment?

_____

*In an emergency, to what hospital would the elderly person be transferred?_____

Will we be notified before the transfer occurs? _____

*If a resident is transferred, for how long will the bed be held? _____

*What is the cost to hold the bed? _____

*Is psychiatric or psychological counseling available? _____

*Is there currently a waiting list?_____ For men?_____ For women? _____

What is the expected waiting period? _____

*Is a deposit required to get on the waiting list? _____

*Are there any circumstances when such a deposit is not refunded?_____

*How often is weight gain or loss monitored? _____

Is it recorded in the medical chart? _____

*How long after admission is the individual care plan prepared? _____

*Once a care plan has been developed, what say do the family and the resident have in its provisions? _____

_____

How is it monitored? _____

How often is it modified? _____

*Who can review the medical chart? _____

*How are families notified about changes in physical or mental condition? _____

*Who makes the decision to change the level of care or transfer the resident to a hospital?

_____

*How are issues of competency in decision making handled? _____

Financial

*Is there a deposit required?_____ *What is the basic monthly fee?_____

When are the bills sent out?_____ By what date must they be paid?_____

Is there a late charge or interest? _____

*Is there an itemized statement of the charges not included in the basic monthly fee?_____

Is it complete?_____

*Are common items excluded that the elderly person will be expected to pay for?_____

_____

How are charges handled that are not on the written statement of extra charges?_____

_____

Can questionable charges be appealed?_____ If so, must they be paid first? _____

Is there an accountant or bookkeeper who can help the elderly person with billing questions or personal matters? _____

Are the facility's books and records audited annually? _____

By whom? _____

Environment

*Is the facility in a convenient location for family and visitors?_____

*Is it easy to access with a wheelchair or walker? _____

*Are there common areas outdoors?_____ *Do they appear safe and secure?_____

*Are the building, grounds, and common areas well-maintained? _____

Is the reception area staffed during all visiting hours to monitor visitors and sign-outs? _____

*What are the visiting hours? _____ Are visiting hours routinely enforced? _____

   *Are children allowed to visit? _____ Are pets allowed to visit? _____

   *Can unwanted visitors be excluded?_____

*Is the facility clean overall? _____

*Are there distinct odors or smells as you enter the facility? _____

*Are the floors carpeted? _____ Are they stained?_____

   *Are wet spots on the floor cleaned up immediately? _____

*Are the bathrooms and bathing areas clean? _____

*Are there grab bars and handrails in the bathrooms and halls? _____

*Are the hallways uncluttered, bright, and easy to navigate? _____

*Is smoking permitted by residents or visitors? _____

Is the indoor temperature comfortable?_____

*Are all doors clearly marked, not just resident doors?_____

   *Are the doors secure? Do they have alarms so residents don't accidentally wander out? _____

Is a floor plan clearly posted?_____

*Are there smoke detectors and sprinklers? _____

*Are exits marked?_____

*Are the public areas—lounges, activity rooms, dining areas—large, warm, and well-lit? _____

*Is the furniture easy for the elderly to get into and out of? _____

*Are signs easy for the elderly to read? _____

Are bulletin boards convenient and readable from a wheelchair? _____

Is everything wheelchair accessible? _____

   If there is an elevator, can a wheelchair-bound person use it alone? _____

   *Are stairs well-lit, with handrails? _____

*Are the rooms bright, airy, and clean? _____

   *Are the beds made? _____

Are bathrooms clearly marked and quickly accessible? _____

*How is privacy assured in a double room? _____

*Are residents dressed with shoes, not just robes and slippers? _____

*Is there evidence of physical restraints? _____

*Are nurse call bells answered promptly? _____

*May residents bring personal possessions? _____

Furniture? _____ Television? _____ Telephone? _____

Are there restrictions or extra charges for clothes or mementos? _____

*How are clothes to be marked? _____

*Who does the resident's personal laundry? _____

*If the facility does the laundry, what does it cost? _____

*How is lost clothing handled? _____

*What is the procedure when personal possessions are lost (dentures, eyeglasses, wedding ring, and so on)? _____

*Has theft been a problem? _____

Is the facility insured or bonded against theft by visitors and staff? _____

How are residents matched when they share a room? _____

*Can residents switch rooms for any reason—roommate, noise, location, assigned staff, and so on?

_____

*Under what conditions will the facility require a resident to move to another room?

_____

May the resident check out of the facility at any time? _____

Meals

*Are residents expected to eat in the dining area? _____

*If so, how many meals? _____ *Are any meals served in the room? _____

*If so, who decides? _____

How is the food kept warm or cold for room meals? _____

When are meals scheduled? _____

    Breakfast_____ Lunch_____ Dinner_____

*Is there a selection of food at each meal? _____

    *Are fresh fruits, vegetables, and dairy products routinely served and available? _____

*Are there extra charges for special meals for dietary or religious reasons? _____

*Can special meal preparation requirements (such as pureed food) be accommodated without extra charges? _____

*Is there a nutritionist or dietitian on staff? _____

    Are nutritional supplements available?_____

*What is the condition of the utensils, plates, and dining room furniture? _____

*Sample the food.

*What is the policy on guests at mealtime? _____

*What snacks are offered and when? _____

Is alcohol permitted? _____

May food be brought into the facility? _____

Is assistance with eating available if needed? _____

Activities

*What activities are routinely planned for residents?_____

*What programs are offered for bedridden patients? _____

*How are these activities designed to meet the residents' physical, emotional, recreational, social, and spiritual needs? _____

*In the last month, how often were activities planned outside the facility? _____

*Is participation voluntary? Is there an extra charge? _____

*How often do community volunteers come into the facility for activities? _____

*Are religious services offered? _____

Support for Residents and Their Families

*Whom can we speak with about the resident council? _____

   *When does the resident council meet? _____

*Is there a family council?_____

   *When does the family council meet? _____

*Who is the contact person for each group?

   Resident council _____

   Family council (if applicable) _____

   How are problems resolved? _____

   *What is the grievance procedure? _____

   *What is the ombudsman's evaluation of the nursing home? _____

   *Are there support groups for residents or family members in the facility? _____

Services Available

*In addition to routine medical services, are these services provided, near or in the facility?

   • Eye care_____

   • Dental care _____

   • Foot care _____

   • Nutritionist services _____

   • Beautician and barber services _____

   • Enteral supplies and products_____

   • Incontinence supplies and products _____

   • Laundry services _____

   • Social service counseling _____

   • Therapy services _____

      • Physical_____

      • Occupational _____

A Family Caregiver's Guide to Planning and Decision Making for the Elderly © 1999 James A. Wilkinson

- Speech _____

- Respiratory _____

- Recreational _____

*Which services cost extra? _____

How are these services paid for?_____

Will the staff arrange the services, if needed? _____

Will any of these services be supplied without the request of the resident, family, or doctor?

_____

Can the family visit the location to see the equipment and meet the staff? _____

Staff

*Is the caregiving staff friendly and courteous toward residents?_____

How does the staff interact with residents? _____

*Is the caregiving staff friendly and courteous toward visitors? _____

*Do residents seem at ease or uncomfortable around staff? _____

*Do the residents appear well cared for? _____

*Does the staff complain about staffing levels or being overworked? _____

If staff members speak another language, do they speak English among themselves in the resident areas? _____

Do staff members belong to a union? _____

What services are routinely performed by volunteers?_____

*If the elderly person would be moving to a particular room, meet the nurses and aides assigned to that room (if any) on at least two shifts.

*How long have those staff members been working there?_____

How far is the elderly person's room from the nurse's station (if applicable)? _____

For Nursing Homes Only

*Medicare-certified? _____

How long certified? _____

How many Medicare beds? _____

*Medicare provider number_____

*Participant in Medicaid program? _____

*Was survey available for review? _____

*Was it posted? _____

*Latest survey date _____

*In the last three years, has the facility received any "A" citations or civil penalties? _____

For what?_____

Was a fine imposed and paid? _____

Is there an RN on each wing on each shift? _____

How many residents does each nurse's aide normally care for on each shift?

Days_____ Evenings_____ Nights _____

*Must a resident be either a private or Medicare resident before he or she can apply for Medicaid?

_____

*Is there someone on staff who will assist in applying for:

Medicare? _____

Medicaid? _____

Third-party insurance? _____

*How are private pay, Medicare deductible, or Medicaid share-of-cost payments billed?

_____

*When are bills sent out?_____ *When are they payable? _____

*Is there a late fee or charge? _____

*How will billing be handled if third-party payment is denied? _____

*Can payments for past months be paid over time?_____

*How are residents' funds handled? _____

How much interest is payable, and how often? _____

A Family Caregiver's Guide to Planning and Decision Making for the Elderly © 1999 James A. Wilkinson

What kind of statements do residents receive? _____

What is the procedure for deposits and withdrawals? _____

*Are facility rules written and posted? _____

*Have an elderlaw attorney or competent adult review the complete admission agreement package.

*Are advance directives requested by the facility? _____

*Will the facility honor the terms of a resident's advance directives?_____

Chapter 6

Advance Directives and Values History

Until recently, when a person went into an irreversible coma, death was expected to quickly follow. Today, modern medicine's ability to keep a person alive for years, even decades, with no regard for his or her quality of life, has led to the creation of advance directives.

What Is an Advance Directive?

The idea of giving instructions that only become effective some time in the future has been around for a long time. Take the will, for example. A will is a legally binding document, completed while a person is alive, that directs how his or her property will be distributed after he or she dies. Three similar legal documents are discussed in this chapter: a general power of attorney, a durable healthcare power of attorney, and a living will.

A power of attorney grants an agent the power to act on behalf of its maker. The person who completes the document is called the "maker" or "principal." The person who receives the power is called the "agent" or "attorney." In this case, "attorney" doesn't mean "lawyer"; it refers to the designated agent, which may be a person or an institution, such as the trust department of a bank.

A general power of attorney is normally used for business and financial matters, such as authorizing someone to sign checks on the maker's behalf. A durable healthcare power of attorney designates someone to make medical decisions on the maker's behalf when he or she cannot. However, while a general power of attorney usually terminates if the maker becomes incompetent, a durable healthcare power of attorney does not. Because a durable healthcare power of attorney lays out the maker's wishes regarding future medical decisions, it is often called an "advance directive."

A living will, another type of advance directive described in this chapter, goes into effect when the person enters an irreversible coma or becomes terminally ill. The living will describes the maker's wishes regarding medical treatment. An agent may or may not be appointed in a living will.

Why Complete an Advance Directive?

The purpose of completing an advance directive is to allow the elderly person to express his or her wishes about future medical care and treatment. The instructions become valid only if the elderly person is unable to make these wishes known (because of stroke, coma, Alzheimer's disease, anesthesia, legal declaration of incompetence, and so forth). It's important to discuss the directive with the elderly person's doctor, clergy, family, and caregivers. The more people who know about an advance directive, the more likely it is to be followed.

Advance directives must be completed in accordance with state law, and the laws vary from state to state. A directive completed in Ohio, for example, may not be effective if the maker moves to Indiana. Because state laws are so rigid, you need a lawyer's input to be sure that the document meets state requirements. Normally, if an advance directive is not completed precisely in accordance with state law, it has no legal power and no one is required to follow it. However, if a family dispute arises over medical care, it could still be used in court as evidence of the person's state of mind at the time it was completed.

Everyone, not just the elderly, should complete an advance directive. There's no way of knowing when an accident, injury, or disease will suddenly deprive us of our decision-making capacity. Without an advance directive, we may lose the right to control our medical care or treatment. And because older adults are particularly prone to injury and disease, it's especially important that they complete an advance directive.

How Does an Advance Directive Work?

Advance directives are based on two basic legal principles: agency and informed consent. Agency is the idea that a competent person has the right to designate someone else to act on his or her behalf. This can be done through a power of attorney. Besides granting someone else the power to act on the maker's behalf, the power of attorney defines what kind of power the agent will have. It could be limited: "To sell my stamp collection to the highest bidder at auction in New York on June 20." Or it could be broad: "To take any action I would take, if I were present." The maker sets the limits, and the agent is free to act within those limits.

According to the legal concept of informed consent, a person has the right to accept or refuse any form of medical care or treatment (except in very limited circumstances), even if the decision could result in his or her death. For example, a Christian Scientist might die because he or she refuses a blood transfusion, but it is his or her right to do so. Furthermore, any proposed medical procedures or treatments must be explained in terms the patient can understand. His or her questions must be answered and the alternatives must be explained.

Advance directives combine these two legal concepts, but what makes an advance directive especially useful is the "durability" of the power. The power is effective even when the maker is no longer competent to make decisions on his or her own.

Personal Values and Beliefs

In addition to completing an advance directive, it's a good idea for the elderly to fill out the *Values History Form* on page 177. It sets forth their views, values, and beliefs about themselves and their medical care, including their feelings and attitudes about treatments, doctors, caregivers, religious beliefs, funeral arrangements, life and personal relationships, and the extent to which their finances should be used to pay for their care. It can inform other people about their wishes concerning invasive tests and surgeries, aggressive intervention to prolong life, organ donation, hospice care, life support, and artificial nutrition or hydration. Although the *Values History Form* is no substitute for an advance directive, it's an invaluable tool to help an agent act in an elderly person's best interests.

It's possible to include values information in an advance directive, but the standard forms don't require it. Furthermore, advance directives need to be read by lawyers, doctors, and family members, and the elderly may not want others to read their most personal thoughts. In cases like these, the elderly person can attach a copy of his or her *Values History Form* to the agent's copy of the advance directive.

Preparing a General Power of Attorney

In a general power of attorney, the maker specifies what kind of power the agent will have, and when the agent can use that power. For example, the maker may grant the agent limited power for a specific period of time—"To sign checks on my behalf during the month of October," for example. In other cases, the power may last until the maker changes the power of attorney or becomes incompetent.

It is possible to make a general power of attorney durable by stating that the power should not terminate if the maker becomes incompetent. Unless the document contains language to make it durable, the power granted to the agent automatically ends when the maker becomes mentally incompetent.

Although a lawyer can tailor the document to fit the maker's wishes, the document generally has four parts:

1. The maker's identity
2. The agent's identity
3. The powers granted to the agent
4. Legal formalities, such as the date and signatures

As already discussed, each state has different requirements, but the following description illustrates what a typical power of attorney form will look like.

Maker's Identity

The first part of the form includes the maker's name and address (or other distinguishing information) and the date the power of attorney becomes effective (usually immediately). It states if the instrument has "springing power," meaning it becomes effective only when some future event occurs, and if it is durable, meaning it continues to be effective until the elderly person's death, regardless of his or her mental competence.

Agent's Identity

The second part of the form appoints an agent, and often an alternate agent in case the first agent can't or won't act. The maker commonly appoints a spouse or close relation as the agent, but if that person's health changes or he or she leaves the family through death or divorce, the alternate agent becomes the primary agent.

The document must specify when responsibilities should shift to an alternate agent. Any ambiguity in this section can create problems later. When problems do arise, if the power isn't durable and there's no question about the elderly person's competence, he or she can just draw up a new power of attorney and revoke the previous one. But if the power is durable and the elderly person has become incompetent, conflicts between the agent and the alternate must usually be resolved through litigation.

Powers Granted

The third part of the form describes the powers granted to the agent, which can be as broad or as narrow as the maker wishes. A power of attorney can be created for a specific act, such as "To sell my house to the highest offer by the end of the year." It can also list in great detail exactly what the agent can or cannot do.

A note of caution: A power of attorney can be drafted to give the agent access to the elderly person's checking account. However, no one should be made a joint signatory on an elderly person's checking account unless there's a very good reason. Legally, this access would transfer ownership of the entire account to that individual, even if this was not the intent. For banking matters, it's better to limit the powers granted.

When you fill out a general power of attorney, the third section might look like this:

I hereby revoke any and all General Powers of Attorney and Special Powers of Attorney that previously have been signed by me. The preceding sentence shall not revoke any Durable Healthcare Power of Attorney or Living Will previously executed by me. Any power granted in this new Power of Attorney shall not confer upon my Agent the authority to act in matters covered by my Durable Healthcare Power of Attorney or Living Will, whether now existing or hereafter created.

I hereby grant to my Agent the power and authority to act on my behalf. This power and authority shall permit my Agent to manage and conduct my affairs and to exercise all of my legal rights and powers, including all rights and powers that I may acquire in the future. My Agent's powers shall include, but not be limited to, the power to:

A. Open, maintain, or close bank accounts (including, but not limited to, checking accounts, savings accounts, and certificates of deposit), brokerage accounts, and other similar accounts with financial institutions.

i. Conduct any business in person or electronically with any financial institution with respect to any of my accounts, including, but not limited to, making deposits and withdrawals, lines of credit, obtaining bank statements, passbooks, drafts, money orders, debit cards, warrants, and certificates or vouchers payable to me by any person, firm, corporation, or political entity.

ii. Perform any act necessary to deposit, negotiate, sell, or transfer any note, security, or draft of the United States of America, any fiscal intermediary of the Medicare program, any state or state agency in connection with the Medicaid program, including any benefit payments (to the extent permitted by applicable law), and any payments from private individuals, corporations, mutual funds, pension funds, or other financial institutions.

iii. Have access to any safe deposit box that I might own, including its contents.

iv. Execute any documents, including powers of attorney on bank-prepared forms, to be able to carry out this power granted.

B. Sell, exchange, buy, invest, or reinvest any assets or property owned by me. Such assets or property may include income-producing or non-income-producing assets and property.

C. Take any and all legal steps necessary to collect any amount or debt owed to me, or to settle any claim, whether made against me or asserted on my behalf against any other person or entity.

D. Enter into binding contracts on my behalf.

E. Exercise all stock rights on my behalf as my proxy, including all rights with respect to stocks, bonds, debentures, or other investments whether held in my name alone or jointly.

F. Sell, convey, lease, mortgage, manage, insure, improve, repair, or perform any other act with respect to any of my property (now owned or later acquired) real or personal, including, but not limited to, the right to remove tenants and to recover possessions). This includes the right to sell or encumber any real or personal property that I now own or may own in the future.

If the Agent is my spouse, then I also hereby appoint _____ as my substitute Agent solely for the purpose of releasing any power or other inchoate interest I might have in any property, including my homestead.

This Power of Attorney shall be construed broadly as a General Power of Attorney. The listing of specific powers is not intended to limit or restrict the general powers granted in this Power of Attorney in any manner.

Any power or authority granted to my Agent under this document shall be limited to the extent necessary to prevent this Power of Attorney from causing:

- my income to be taxable to my Agent,
- my assets to be subject to a general power of appointment by my Agent, and

• my Agent to have any incidents of owner-ship with respect to any life insurance poli-cies that I may own on the life of my Agent.

This section of a general power of attorney might also contain provisions that

- Protect the agent from liability if he or she has taken actions in good faith.
- Authorize payment to the agent for his or her services.
- Require the agent to account for every action he or she takes.
- Allow the document to be revoked automat-ically if a new power of attorney is created.

If the document includes a provision that makes it a durable power, there may also be a section explaining how the elderly person wishes it to interact with any advance directives:

This Power of Attorney shall become effective imme-diately, and shall not be affected by my disability or lack of mental competence, except as may be pro-vided otherwise by an applicable state statute. This is a Durable Power of Attorney. This Power of Attorney shall continue to be effective until my death.

No power granted herein shall interfere or be deemed inconsistent with any authority granted by me in a document titled Durable Healthcare Power of Attorney, whether such document is executed before or after the date of this document. Notwithstanding any other provision of this Power of Attorney, it is my intent that my Agent have no authority to interfere or become involved with any matter involving my med-ical care or treatment, the provision of medical ser-vices or products, or decisions to forego or withdraw medical treatments.

Legal Formalities

The last part of the power of attorney form includes all the elements needed to make it a binding legal document, such as the date, the elderly person's signature, the witnesses' signatures, notarization, and a "prepared by" statement. The form may need to be notarized and recorded with the local record-ing office, especially if the powers granted include the right to buy, sell, or lease real property.

Preparing a Durable Healthcare Power of Attorney

Unlike most powers of attorney, which usually go into effect immediately, a durable healthcare power of attorney may take effect immediately or not until the maker becomes legally incompetent.

When drawing up a durable healthcare power of attorney, keep the following points in mind:

1. A durable healthcare power of attorney can only be made while the elderly person is legally competent. If an elderly person is no longer competent, he or she can no longer create a durable healthcare power of attorney—or any power of attorney, for that matter. If there's any

question about the person's competency, or if a dispute over competency is likely to result, seek a lawyer's advice. The lawyer may advise you to get a written opinion from a doctor regarding the elderly person's mental state. He or she might also suggest that you create a record (often a video-taped interview) of the elderly person discussing and executing the documents. This will show that the person is aware of his or her surroundings and understands his or her actions.

2. Legally competent people are free to make their own choices about medical care,

even if others think they've made the wrong decision. A mentally competent person is free to choose death over a potentially life-saving procedure, such as CPR, even if a doctor disagrees with the decision. Although family members may fervently believe that all means should be used to keep the person alive, a durable healthcare power of attorney may direct the agent not to authorize CPR under any circumstances.

3. A durable healthcare power of attorney is effective only when the elderly person is unable to give informed consent. A durable healthcare power of attorney is effective any time the elderly person cannot give informed consent (when under anesthesia, for example), and it ceases to be effective when and if he or she becomes competent again. This is different from a living will (page 174), which normally takes effect only when the elderly person becomes terminally ill or irreversibly unconscious.

4. Because a durable healthcare power of attorney becomes effective when a person becomes legally incompetent, it's important to know when that point is reached. If state law has a procedure for determining when a durable healthcare power of attorney takes effect, it must be followed exactly, and this may involve both doctors and attorneys. If state law is silent on this point, then the document itself should explain, in detail, the point at which the power will take effect. This ensures that the elderly person knows and approves of the procedure that will be used to determine his or her competency.

5. A durable healthcare power of attorney grants power to a specific person to act in the elderly person's best interests. A durable healthcare power of attorney is flexible—it gives the agent the authority to make decisions as events unfold. Take the example of a woman who designated her sister as her agent. During surgery, a complication arose that required a procedure the woman hadn't been asked about or given consent to beforehand. The durable healthcare power of attorney allowed the sister to give the surgeon permission to proceed with the operation. Once the woman recovered, she began making her own healthcare decisions again.

A durable healthcare power of attorney also helps eliminate confusion about who can give consent. In this case, the woman's sister had the power to decide—not her husband, children, or other siblings. A medical dilemma was speedily resolved and a potential family conflict avoided.

6. Each state has different laws to regulate the durable healthcare power of attorney form. The durable healthcare power of attorney is carefully regulated in most states. Some states have a specific form that must be used, whereas others have a "suggested" form. In some states, certain provisions ("magic words") must be included to make it durable; in others, only witnesses and signatures are required. Because the laws vary, you must consult an elderlaw attorney to be sure all the legal requirements are met.

In addition, the name of the form will vary from state to state. Some states will call it a durable healthcare power of attorney, others will call it a healthcare proxy, and so forth. When speaking with a lawyer, focus on what you're trying to accomplish instead of the name of the form you think you might need. You might also contact Choice in Dying (page 235). For a nominal fee, this organization will forward the proper state forms to you.

The Aging with Dignity web site (page 255) has a durable healthcare power of attorney—called The Five Wishes form—that you can download for free. While it is not valid in every state, it is a good place to start when thinking about your wishes for future medical care.

7. A living will is different from a durable healthcare power of attorney, although both documents may be combined on one form. A living will specifies which medical procedures the elderly person wishes to have done, or not to have done, if he or she becomes terminally ill or enters an irreversible coma. A durable healthcare power of attorney, on the other hand, allows an agent to make healthcare decisions on the elderly person's behalf anytime he or she becomes incompetent.

It's possible to combine a living will (page 174) with a durable healthcare power of attorney and execute both documents at once. In this case, the agent is permitted to act in circumstances where a living will would not apply.

A durable healthcare power of attorney form looks similar to a general power of attorney. Like the general power of attorney, the durable healthcare power of attorney document has four parts—the maker, the agent, the powers granted, and the legal requirements. Unlike the general power of attorney, the durable healthcare power of attorney may include a "living will" provision.

Maker's Identity

The first part of the form identifies the elderly person, indicates when the power is to become effective, and states that it is durable. While a durable healthcare power of attorney usually doesn't become effective until the elderly person becomes legally incompetent, it can be drafted to be effective immediately, which bypasses any questions about the onset of incompetence.

Agent's Identity

The second part appoints the agent, as well as one or more alternate agents. There are three main reasons for appointing alternate agents:

1. In an emergency, the primary agent may be unreachable. Depending on the elderly person's medical condition, it may not be possible or desirable to wait for the agent to turn up.

2. In the case of emotionally charged issues, such as ending life support or using aggressive procedures to keep the person alive, the agent (often the elderly person's spouse) may be unable to make a rational decision and will therefore refuse to do anything.

3. When the time comes, the agent (again, often a spouse) may have deteriorated mentally and may no longer be competent enough to make decisions. He or she may be unable to understand the medical issues well enough to give consent.

If the elderly person chooses not to appoint a series of alternate agents, he or she may draft the durable healthcare power of attorney so that the primary agent can appoint a new agent, if necessary. (This is seldom done for a general power of attorney, because the elderly person can just appoint someone else.) The elderly person can require the new agent to be someone who knows him or her and is familiar with his or her beliefs and wishes.

This section also includes the agent's address, as well as any telephone numbers, e-mail addresses, and fax numbers. Listing as many ways to reach the agent as possible will help the caregiver or medical personnel contact the agent in a medical emergency.

Powers Granted

The third area of the durable healthcare power of attorney—powers granted—lists all the powers that the agent will have. This section is normally shorter in a durable healthcare power of attorney than in a general power of attorney. It might read:

A. To authorize, withhold, or withdraw medical care or surgical procedures;

B. To authorize, withhold, or withdraw nutrition (food) or hydration (water) medically supplied by tube through my nose, stomach, intestine, or veins;

C. To authorize my admission or discharge from a medical, nursing, residential, or similar facility and to make arrangements or contacts for my care, including home healthcare, home care, or hospice care;

D. To have full access to my medical and hospital records and all information regarding my physical and mental health, and to be able to discuss any aspect of my care with my doctors or others to be able to give informed consent;

E. To make an anatomical gift of all or part of my body;

F. To hire and fire medical, home care, social service, and other personnel who support or provide my medical or personal care; and

G. To take any legal action necessary to carry out my wishes as expressed in this Durable Healthcare Power of Attorney or as my Agent believes are in my best interests in connection with my medical care or treatment.

An alternative, which in many respects is even broader, might read:

My Agent is authorized to make any and all healthcare decisions for me that my Agent may be called upon to make or as deemed appropriate by my Agent, based upon my Agent's understanding of my situation and subject to my wishes and any limitations otherwise set forth in this instrument. A "healthcare decision" is an informed decision to accept, maintain, condition, discontinue, or refuse any care, treatment, intervention, service, or procedure to maintain, diagnose, or treat my physical or mental condition.

My Agent shall request and evaluate information concerning my medical condition, diagnosis, prognosis, and the risks and benefits of any proposed medical treatment; the provision, withholding, or withdrawal of any personal care, medical procedure, or service to maintain, diagnose, treat, or provide for my physical or mental health.

My Agent will consider the decision that I would have made if I had the ability to do so. If my Agent does not know my wishes regarding a specific healthcare decision, my Agent shall make a decision in what my Agent determines are my best interests. In considering my best interests, my Agent shall consider my personal beliefs and values to the extent known by my Agent from any source.

Living Will Provision

If state law permits, and if the elderly person wishes to include it, this section can also contain a "living will" provision, directing healthcare professionals and the agent to act in a certain way if the elderly person becomes terminally ill or permanently unconscious. In some situations, the elderly person may also wish to include a statement about his or her goals or philosophy to assist the agent in making decisions (see Values History on page 176). It's unlikely that the agent and the maker will discuss every possible situation that could arise, so a few general statements could help the agent determine what treatment the elderly person would want if the living will provision does not expressly cover it. Also, if the question of ending life support ever arises, a statement from the elderly person about this issue may help the agent make the decision.

The living will provision might include any (but not all) of the following general statements:

• I want my life prolonged to the greatest extent possible, without regard to my condition, my chances for recovery or survival, or the cost of the treatment or procedure.

• If I have an incurable or terminal illness, injury, or condition with no reasonable hope of long-term recovery or survival, I do not want life-sustaining procedures or treatments to be used.

• If the costs of treatment to be provided or continued outweigh the expected benefits, I do not want life-sustaining treatments to be used. My Agent is to consider the possible relief from suffering, the preservation and restoration of functioning, and the quality of my life if extended.

• Upon admission to any healthcare facility, I want my Agent to decline the use of cardiac resuscitation and mechanical respiration under all circumstances. If the healthcare facility will not agree in advance to honor such a request, I do not want to be admitted there.

• Due to my religious beliefs, I do not want my Agent to consent to or permit the use of any blood or blood products, even if necessary to save or prolong my life.

• If my organs can be donated, it is my wish that they be used in the best way possible to help others. If they are not suitable for donation to others, my wish is that they be used in research. Any steps that are necessary to preserve the organs for donation may be consented to by my Agent.

• If my Agent is informed by two or more medical personnel that I am capable of feeling pain or discomfort due to my medical condition, it is my wish that my Agent consent to any healthcare treatment to relieve pain or to provide comfort, even if such treatment might shorten my life, suppress my appetite or breathing, or be habit forming.

• If my Agent is not sure what decision I might have made in a given situation, my Agent should decide what he or she believes is in my best interest, recognizing that this could mean permitting my death even though life could be sustained through extraordinary means.

The maker might decide not to make any statements, leaving everything up to the agent's discretion. On the other hand, he or she might include directions or limitations that are even more specific than those just listed.

If you're not sure what a provision in a state-mandated form means, or if you don't know how to express a concern, direction, or belief in a legal document, consult your doctor, lawyer, family, or clergy.

The living will provision might conclude with two statements:

_____ My Agent must follow these instructions, or

_____ These instructions are only to assist the Agent, but, after considering the precise facts and circumstances when a decision has to be made, my Agent has the authority to override my instructions.

On behalf of myself, my executors, and my heirs, I hold my Agent or Agents and all my healthcare providers harmless, and release and indemnify them against any claim for recognizing my Agent's or Agents' authority or for following my instructions in good faith.

Legal Formalities

The last part of a durable healthcare power of attorney includes signatures, witnesses, and so forth, which must be completed in accordance with state law. An attorney will know exactly how to format this section. It is critical that no mistakes be made or the form will be legally void. Be especially cautious about using preprinted forms out of books or magazines without seeking the advice of a lawyer and following his or her directions exactly.

Preparing a Living Will

A living will normally goes into effect when a person enters an irreversible coma or becomes terminally ill with no hope of recovery. Normally, a living will does not appoint an agent or grant any discretionary power; it simply lays out the maker's wishes about what medical treatment, if any, should occur from that point on. Keep in mind the following:

1. It's important to distinguish between brain death and irreversible coma. In both cases, a respirator or ventilator is used to keep the patient breathing. However, once the brain has ceased functioning, the person is considered brain dead and the legal definition of death has been met; there is no hope of recovery. At this point, a living will and any powers of attorney are no longer in effect. When a person is brain dead, the hospital may keep the respirator going until the family makes a decision about organ donation, but this only preserves the person's organs; it has nothing to do with keeping him or her alive.

If brain death has not occurred, the person is considered alive even if he or she is not expected to recover. If the person has a living will, this will direct the medical care or treatment he or she receives until brain death occurs. In some cases, brain death may occur within hours; in other cases, within years.

2. If a person has both a durable healthcare power of attorney and a living will, there may be confusion about which should apply. A living will may be drafted as part of a durable healthcare power of attorney (to tell the agent how to act if a terminal condition develops) or on a separate state-approved form. If the elderly person creates both a living will and a durable healthcare power of attorney, it may contain conflicting information. For example, the elderly person may want CPR, but only if there's hope for recovery.

As a result, the power of attorney might require it, and the living will could prohibit it.

Rather than have two separate documents, it may be a good idea to have only a durable healthcare power of attorney. If state law permits, a durable healthcare power of attorney may include detailed instructions that would otherwise be found in a living will. This would not only eliminate confusion about which document should apply, but also give the agent some authority to take circumstances (the patient's likelihood of recovery, and so forth) into account when making a healthcare decision.

3. A living will can give specific, although limited, directions for treatment. Anyone preparing a living will must confront this question: If death is certain and there is no reasonable hope of recovery, how much medical intervention do I want to keep me alive (in the legal sense)? There are basically two options: "Do nothing to keep me alive, and stop whatever you are doing now," or "Do everything to keep me alive, no matter how ineffective or expensive it might be."

Most living will forms have some general provisions, such as the following:

I direct my doctor to withhold or withdraw life-sustaining treatment that serves only to prolong the process of dying, and to provide treatment only to keep me comfortable and to relieve pain, including pain that may occur by withholding or withdrawing life-sustaining treatment, even if that treatment might shorten my life, be habit forming, or suppress my appetite.

If my doctor believes that a particular life-sustaining provision may lead to a significant recovery, I direct my doctor to implement the treatment for a reasonable period of time. If it does not significantly improve my condition, I direct that the treatment be withdrawn even if it shortens my life.

Whether you're using a state-mandated form or a form prepared by an attorney, you may be able to expressly request or refuse specific procedures. Here are some examples from the Pennsylvania state form:

I [ ] do [ ] do not want cardiac resuscitation.
I [ ] do [ ] do not want mechanical respiration.
I [ ] do [ ] do not want tube feeding or any other artificial or invasive form of nutrition (food) or hydration (water).
I [ ] do [ ] do not want blood or blood products.
I [ ] do [ ] do not want any form of surgery or invasive diagnostic tests.
I [ ] do [ ] do not want kidney dialysis.
I [ ] do [ ] do not want antibiotics.

I realize that if I do not specifically indicate my preference regarding any of the forms of treatment listed above, I may receive that form of treatment.

Notice that this last sentence goes against the notion of informed consent. If the person were legally competent, none of these procedures could be done without his or her permission. However, when a person is in an irreversible coma with no reasonable hope of recovery and without having given specific instructions to proceed, medical procedures may be performed without consent, no matter how futile, expensive, or unreasonable.

Before choosing which medical procedures the living will would require or prohibit, the elderly person must understand what is involved in the procedure, as well as its expected outcome, its invasiveness, its cost, and the alternatives (including death). For example, most studies indicate that cardiac resuscitation on the frail elderly will usually fail unless undertaken immediately and in an acute care hospital. If it's successful, the elderly person will probably have brain damage, broken ribs and teeth, and chronic pain from the resuscitation effort. Before including cardiac resuscitation in the living will, the elderly person needs to decide if this is the kind of life to which he or she wants to be resuscitated.

A living will may designate an agent or surrogate decision maker. However, it's not always necessary to appoint an agent. If the elderly person has given comprehensive instructions, there would be little for an agent to decide. Furthermore, if a durable healthcare power of attorney exists, there will already be an agent designated to act on the elderly person's behalf. On the other hand, if the elderly person has only expressed a general intent in the living will and hasn't prepared a durable healthcare power of attorney, it may be best to appoint an agent.

Values History: Helping the Elderly Make Their Wishes Known

The following information has been adapted from the *Values History Form,* published by the Center for Health, Law, and Ethics at the University of New Mexico School of Law.

What You Need to Know

The *Values History Form* is not a legal document, but it can be used to supplement a living will or durable healthcare power of attorney. This form is not copyrighted; you're encouraged to make copies for friends and relatives to use.

The *Values History Form* recognizes that our medical decisions are based on beliefs and values: How do we feel about control and independence? About pain, illness, dying, and death? What gives us pleasure? What gives us sorrow? This is valuable information for anyone who might someday have to make medical decisions on our behalf. By informing friends and family of our wishes, we can reduce family conflicts and lessen the burden of their responsibility.

How to Use the *Values History Form*

The *Values History Form* discusses a number of issues, such as an individual's:

- Attitude toward his or her health
- Feelings about healthcare providers
- Thoughts about independence and control
- Personal relationships

- Attitude toward life
- Attitude toward illness, dying, and death
- Religious background and beliefs
- Preferences about living environment
- Attitude toward finances
- Wishes for a funeral

Have the elderly person answer the questions listed on the *Values History Form.* He or she might write out thoughts ahead of time, or bring together family and friends to discuss each question. Feel free to add your own questions and comments to those already provided.

It's easier to talk about these issues before a medical crisis occurs, but if that's not possible, making copies of the *Values History Form* and handing them out to others may be enough to get them talking about a painful and difficult subject.

Make sure that everyone who might be involved in future medical decisions is aware of the elderly person's wishes.

While it's essential for the elderly to prepare a *Values History Form,* it's just as important for younger people to discuss these issues and make their wishes known. In fact, some of the most difficult medical decisions are made on behalf of younger patients. If the patient has already shared his or her wishes with family and friends, the decision makers might have more peace of mind.

VALUES HISTORY FORM

Name_____

Date_____

If someone assisted you in completing this form, please fill in his or her name, address, and relationship to you.

Name_____

Address _____

_____

Relationship _____

It's important that your medical treatment be your choice.

The purpose of this form is to assist you in thinking about and writing down what is important to you about your health. If you should at some time become unable to make healthcare decisions, this form may help others make a decision for you in accordance with your values.

The first section of this form provides an opportunity for you to discuss your values, wishes, and preferences in a number of different areas such as your personal relationships, your overall attitude toward life, and your thoughts about illness.

The second section of this form provides a space for indicating whether you have completed an Advance Directive, e.g. a Living Will, Durable Power of Attorney for Healthcare Decisions or Advance Directive for Healthcare, and where these documents may be found.

This form is not copyrighted; you may make as many copies as you wish.

This form was developed by the Center for Health, Law, and Ethics, Institute of Public Law, University of New Mexico School of Law, 1117 Stanford N.E., Albuquerque, New Mexico 87131.

OVERALL ATTITUDE TOWARD LIFE AND HEALTH

What would you like to say to someone reading this document about your overall attitude toward life?

_____

_____

_____

_____

_____

What goals do you have for the future?

_____

_____

_____

_____

How satisfied are you with what you have achieved in your life?

_____

_____

_____

_____

What, for you, makes life worth living?

_____

_____

_____

_____

What do you fear most? What frightens or upsets you?

_____

_____

_____

_____

What activities do you enjoy (e.g., hobbies, watching TV, etc.)?

_____

_____

_____

_____

How would you describe your current state of health?

_____

_____

_____

_____

If you currently have any health problems or disabilities, how do they affect: you? your family? your work? your ability to function?

_____

_____

_____

_____

If you have any health problems or disabilities, how do you feel about them? What would you like others (family, friends, doctors) to know about this?

_____

_____

_____

_____

Do you have difficulties in getting through the day with activities such as: eating? preparing food? sleeping? dressing and bathing? etc.

_____

_____

_____

_____

What would you say to someone reading this document about your general health?

_____

_____

_____

_____

PERSONAL RELATIONSHIPS

What role do family and friends play in your life?

_____

_____

_____

_____

How do you expect friends, family, and others to support your decisions regarding medical treatment you may need now or in the future?

_____

_____

_____

_____

Have you made any arrangements for family or friends to make medical treatment decisions on your behalf? If so, who has agreed to make decisions for you and in what circumstances?

_____

_____

_____

_____

What general comments would you like to make about the personal relationships in your life?

_____

_____

_____

_____

THOUGHTS ABOUT INDEPENDENCE AND SELF-SUFFICIENCY

How does independence or dependence affect your life?

_____

_____

_____

_____

If you were to experience decreased physical and mental abilities, how would that affect your attitude toward independence and self-sufficiency?

_____

_____

_____

_____

If your current physical or mental health gets worse, how would you feel?

_____

_____

_____

_____

LIVING ENVIRONMENT

Have you lived alone or with others over the past ten years?

_____

_____

_____

_____

How comfortable have you been in your surroundings? How might illness, disability, or age affect this?

_____

_____

_____

_____

What general comments would you like to make about your surroundings?

_____

_____

_____

_____

RELIGIOUS BACKGROUND AND BELIEFS

What is your spiritual/religious background?

_____

_____

_____

_____

How do your beliefs affect your feelings toward serious, chronic, or terminal illness?

_____

_____

_____

_____

How does your faith community, church, or synagogue support you?

_____

_____

What general comments would you like to make about your beliefs?

_____

_____

_____

_____

RELATIONSHIPS WITH DOCTORS AND OTHER CAREGIVERS

How do you relate to your doctors? Please comment on: trust; decision making; time for satisfactory communication; respectful treatment.

_____

_____

_____

_____

How do you feel about other caregivers, including nurses, therapists, chaplains, social workers, etc.?

_____

_____

_____

_____

What else would you like to say about doctors and other caregivers?

_____

_____

_____

_____

THOUGHTS ABOUT ILLNESS, DYING, AND DEATH

What general comments would you like to make about illness, dying, and death?

_____

_____

_____

_____

What will be important to you when you are dying (e.g., physical comfort, no pain, family members present, etc.)?

_____

_____

_____

_____

Where would you prefer to die?

_____

_____

_____

_____

How do you feel about the use of life-sustaining measures if you were: suffering from an irreversible chronic illness (e.g., Alzheimer's disease)? terminally ill? in a permanent coma?

_____

_____

_____

_____

What general comments would you like to make about medical treatment?

_____

_____

_____

_____

FINANCES

What general comments would you like to make about your finances and the cost of healthcare?

_____

_____

_____

_____

What are your feelings about having enough money to provide for your care?

_____

_____

_____

_____

FUNERAL PLANS

What general comments would you like to make about your funeral and burial or cremation?

_____

_____

_____

_____

Have you made your funeral arrangements? If so, with whom?

_____

_____

_____

OPTIONAL QUESTIONS

How would you like your obituary (announcement of your death) to read?

_____

_____

_____

_____

Write yourself a brief eulogy (a statement about yourself to be read at your funeral).

_____

_____

_____

_____

What would you like to say to someone reading this *Values History Form?*

_____

_____

_____

_____

LEGAL DOCUMENTS

What legal documents about healthcare decisions have you signed?

Living will? _____ Yes _____ No

If yes, where can it be found? Name, address, and phone number.

_____

_____

_____

Durable Power of Attorney for Healthcare Decisions? _____ Yes _____ No

If yes, where can it be found? Name, address, and phone number.

_____

_____

_____

_____

Advance Directive for Healthcare? _____ Yes _____ No

If yes, where can it be found? Name, address, and phone number.

_____

_____

_____

_____

Other? _____ Yes _____ No

If yes, where can it be found? Name, address, and phone number.

_____

_____

_____

_____

Chapter 7

Resources

Choosing Professionals

One of the main goals of this book is to help you gather information so you can make informed decisions about caring for the elderly. While caregiving decisions are usually made by the elderly person, the caregiver, or the family, there are occasions when professional advice may be necessary. This section discusses several kinds of professionals who can assist the elderly and their caregivers. Please note that professionals who supply home healthcare, home care, and housekeeping services are not discussed here; they are covered fully in chapter 4.

Doctors and Clergy

Although doctors and clergy provide very different services, they have one thing in common—the elderly tend to establish relationships with these professionals early in life, and these relationships often continue into old age.

When they need medical attention, most elderly people want to see their doctor. They're not inclined to switch, even if they're not particularly happy with the care they receive. If an elderly person has developed a long-term relationship with a doctor, the caregiver shouldn't upset this relationship unless he or she believes a change in doctors is necessary. If the elderly person must switch primary care doctors, the caregiver should try to find a board-certified gerontologist. If there isn't one available, a family practitioner or internist should be sought.

The relationship between an elderly person and his or her rabbi, priest, or minister can have a profound effect on his or her well-being. The clergy's willingness to make home and nursing home visits, to counsel families, to address issues of death and dying, and to involve the elderly in a spiritual community are all important aspects of caregiving. Although these relationships tend to carry over from earlier years, they are more often tied to a particular church, mosque, or synagogue than to a particular person. If the church gets a new minister, the elderly person does, too.

If you hear of a member of the clergy who specializes in ministering to the elderly, you might consider introducing him or her to the elderly person, even if he or she isn't of the same religion.

Geriatric Care Managers

The term "geriatric care manager" refers to a trained professional who is knowledgeable about community services available to the elderly and can arrange to have these services provided.

Geriatric care managers are sometimes called "professional care managers."

Many care managers are members of the National Association of Professional Geriatric Care Managers. Membership in this organization is a sign of quality, because members must demonstrate their competence before they're allowed to join. Other than this, there are few standards one must meet before calling oneself a geriatric care manager.

Generally, professional care managers agree to provide specific services in exchange for a fixed fee, which ranges from $50 to $175 per hour. (Social workers and discharge planners may provide these services as well, and are often less expensive.) The cost is usually paid by the person who hires the care manager, although it is sometimes covered by insurance. In fact, more and more companies are making this benefit available so their employees can provide long-distance caregiving without having to take extended leaves of absence.

There are three main reasons to consider hiring a geriatric care manager:

1. The long-distance caregiver needs another pair of eyes to assist the elderly person at home or to assure that appropriate care is being provided.

2. The family isn't familiar with the resources in the community or doesn't believe they can choose a competent provider without professional help.

3. Geriatric assessment or testimony may be needed for a court incompetency hearing.

When selecting a geriatric care manager, focus on his or her background, experience, and accreditation. Don't hesitate to ask for references—the best references are from families who have used the care manager's services and from professionals in the community, such as elderlaw attorneys, hospital discharge planners, and gerontologists. For a more detailed discussion about selecting care managers, read chapter 4.

Your contract with a geriatric care manager should specify the frequency of service, fees involved, terms of payment, and name of the person supplying the service. Professional care managers may not perform all the services themselves, and they might end up providing some services that aren't included in the base rate. Therefore, the arrangement needs to be clearly understood at the outset. Although some professional care managers might disagree, it may be best to look for geriatric care managers who provide consulting services only. If they begin to supply products and services through their own companies, their independence and objectivity become compromised.

Financial Planners

In recent years, the need for financial planning has risen dramatically among the elderly. Many elderly people are living either on reduced survivor's benefits or on pension and Social Security income, which are essentially fixed at around age sixty-two. Furthermore, longer life expectancy can further stretch limited financial resources.

You will need to hire a financial planner:

• if you have concerns about how the elderly person is managing his or her affairs, or

• if, after completing the *Vital Information Form* (pages 9–33) and *Financial Worksheets* (pages 39–54), you realize that either the elderly person's affairs need to be managed differently or previous mismanagement means that finances must be straightened out. (The goal should be to preserve assets, not to maximize returns.)

You may encounter several types of planners, including certified public accountants (CPAs), certified life underwriters (CLUs), and certified financial planners (CFPs). CPAs have strong accounting and tax backgrounds, CLUs tend to be more experienced with insurance matters, and CFPs have a broad background in a range of financial planning areas. Although there are many acceptable, safe investment alternatives, be careful when a CLU recommends life insurance or a CFP suggests a product for which he or she will receive a large commission.

Stockbrokers, too, are routinely classified as financial advisers. However, their compensation is based largely on trading activity in stocks, bonds, and mutual funds. Therefore, they tend to give advice that will result in trades. While this advice can be beneficial, it points to a conflict of interest. Bank employees also may be able to offer investment advice, but they might have a conflict of interest as well. When choosing a financial planner, it may be best to avoid individuals who receive a commission or other financial incentive from someone else if you follow their advice.

In recent years, many accounting and brokerage firms have hired tax and estate planning attorneys and CFPs to advise clients. If you choose to get advice from a corporation, find out who is providing the advice and what his or her credentials are.

When selecting a financial planner, it is critical to look at his or her experience, reputation, qualifications, and credentials. Furthermore, if the planner is to make investment suggestions, he or she must be registered with the Securities and Exchange Commission (SEC). The International Association for Financial Planning's Customer Referral Program (page 227) can send you information on potential advisers, including their education, expertise, designations, and experience.

This area is rife with fraud. Never hire advisers without independently verifying their reputation and credentials, especially if you're investing in a product or service for which they will receive a commission. Find out how the planners are compensated. Ask them for references—preferably from people you know—and check them. Find out if they work with local professionals, such as accountants, lawyers, or insurance agents. Find out if they routinely deal with the elderly and what their area of specialty is. Know what they charge, who will actually do the work, and what services will be provided.

Lawyers

Like relationships with doctors and clergy, legal relationships tend to carry over from an elderly person's earlier years. However, unless an attorney is well-versed in elderlaw, his or her advice can lead to devastating consequences for the elderly person and the caregiver. Elderlaw is a specialized area. Many competent and experienced attorneys simply don't understand the issues that might arise. If the elderly person does not have an attorney, get references from friends and other caregivers to find a good elderlaw attorney in your area. If the elderly person is comfortable with a particular attorney, perhaps that attorney will recognize his or her limitations and recommend an elderlaw specialist. It's worth asking.

Because the legal profession has no uniform standards to determine competence in specific areas, you must use caution when choosing an elderlaw attorney. Remember, competence in one area of the law does not imply competence in another. Furthermore, attorneys can say they practice elderlaw, join the local bar association's elderlaw section, and claim to be an elderlaw expert—yet be totally unqualified. Finally, although large law firms tend to have good lawyers, often their size and cost structure make it difficult for them to practice elderlaw effectively. Elderlaw is as much about listening and counseling as it is about providing legal advice or complicated documents. At $250 per hour, listening and caring become quite expensive.

When choosing an elderlaw attorney:

1. Look for someone who specializes in elderlaw (or estate planning, if that's what you need)

and who understands third-party reimbursement (especially Medicaid planning), advance directives, and the rights of the elderly.

2. Look for someone who can advocate for the elderly person.

3. Understand the attorney's fee structure and payment expectations, and be sure to check references.

4. Find out how much of the attorney's time is actually spent practicing elderlaw.

5. Observe how he or she interacts with the elderly person and assess his or her counseling skills.

6. Make sure he or she is familiar with trusts and estate planning, durable healthcare powers of attorney, and home care contracting.

7. Perhaps most importantly, assess how the attorney attempts to gain the trust and confidence of the elderly person.

Collecting Key Documents

A recurrent theme throughout this book has been the importance of collecting key documents before you need them. This section provides a *Document Checklist* (a comprehensive list of the documents you should try to collect) as well as a *Document Collection Form* (space to record important information about each document). These documents should be kept in a safe place where they are readily accessible. You will need to make copies of the *Document Collection Form* (beginning on page 197)—as well as some of the documents themselves—and give them to family members and the elderly person's lawyer.

Use the *Document Checklist* to gather the documents you need before filling out the *Document Collection Form*. Collecting these documents may be difficult. Some may be inaccessible; others you simply won't be able to find. Also, the elderly person might not want you to see certain documents, such as his or her last will and testament. If you can't get copies of a document, but you know that it exists, try to find out the date it was prepared and the location of the original.

There are three main reasons for collecting documents:

1. To create an up-to-date checklist of important documents so you know which you have and which you are missing.

2. To make sure that the documents are protected against accidental (or intentional) destruction.

3. To tell you exactly where vital documents are in case they are needed.

In general, the *Document Collection Form* needs to be updated whenever a vital document changes. However, some documents, such as checking account statements and federal tax returns, will change frequently. In cases like these, the date of the document isn't as important as establishing the existence of a legal relationship. A checking account is a good example. It's more important to know the name of the bank, the account number, and the authorized signers on the account than it is to know the latest balance. You don't need to update the *Document Collection Form* each time you get a new bank statement, but if the elderly person changes banks, you should note this and get copies of the new documents.

The *Document Collection Form* is intended to be comprehensive. The elderly person likely won't have a need for every document on the list. Even if you think an item doesn't apply, however, it's best to ask. If the item doesn't apply, write "NA" on the first line. Naturally, if you don't understand an item on the list, ask an attorney what it means or why it might be important.

Three significant items aren't included on the list:

1. The forms you've completed throughout this book. Copies of these forms should be kept with your documents from the *Document Collection Form*.

2. Passwords and access codes. While it's important to know the passwords and access codes for home security systems, ATM machines, and e-mail accounts, you don't want others to have access to this information.

3. Keys. Be sure to make copies of the car keys, house or apartment keys, post office box key, and safety deposit box key. Keep them in one place so you can get to them in an emergency.

The items on the *Document Collection Form* are numbered, so if you need to continue on a separate sheet of paper, you can reference the correct document.

DOCUMENT CHECKLIST

_____ 1. Adoption papers

_____ 2. Annuity policies

_____ 3. Automobile titles or leases

_____ 4. Balance statements (checking, savings, Christmas Club, IRA, 401(k), 403(b), Keogh, credit union, money market, lines of credit, and so on)

_____ 5. Baptism records

_____ 6. Bar/Bat Mitzvah records

_____ 7. Birth certificate

_____ 8. Bonds (not held in brokerage account)

_____ 9. Brokerage statements (stocks, bonds, mutual funds, and so on)

_____ 10. Citizenship/naturalization papers

_____ 11. Credit/debit cards

_____ 12. Death certificate of spouse (or prior spouse)

_____ 13. Deeds to real property

_____ 14. Deferred compensation agreements

_____ 15. Divorce decree, settlement agreements, and court orders

_____ 16. Driver's license

_____ 17. Employment history

_____ 18. Funeral/cremation, prepaid funeral, cemetery plot, organ donation

_____ 19. Gift tax returns (federal and state)

_____ 20. Group health booklets and ID cards

_____ 21. Group life policies, certificates, booklets

_____ 22. Income tax returns (federal, state, and local) for the last seven years

_____ 23. Inheritance documents

_____ 24. Inventory of possessions in the home

_____ 25. Investment club agreement

_____ 26. Last will and testament, including codicils

_____ 27. Legal claims as plaintiff, defendant, or class member

A Family Caregiver's Guide to Planning and Decision Making for the Elderly © 1999 James A. Wilkinson

_____ 28. Life insurance policies, certificates of insurance

_____ 29. Living will

_____ 30. Loans or debts due to the elderly person

_____ 31. Loans or debts owed by the elderly person

_____ 32. Long-term care insurance policy, booklet

_____ 33. Marriage certificate

_____ 34. Medicaid beneficiary ID

_____ 35. Medicare ID

_____ 36. Membership list

_____ 37. Military discharge certificate

_____ 38. Mortgages for each property

_____ 39. Mortgage insurance

_____ 40. Organ donor card

_____ 41. Partnerships (general and limited)

_____ 42. Passport

_____ 43. Pension or retirement plans (booklets, statements, benefit summaries, retiree health)

_____ 44. Personal address book

_____ 45. Personal contracts

_____ 46. Pet information

_____ 47. Powers of attorney (durable healthcare)

_____ 48. Powers of attorney (general or special)

_____ 49. Prenuptial or postnuptial agreement

_____ 50. Prescription drug plans (ID cards, booklet)

_____ 51. Property and casualty insurance.

_____ 52. Property and school tax receipts from the past three years.

_____ 53. Rental/time share agreements

_____ 54. Safety deposit box and home safe contents

_____ 55. Savings bonds

_____ 56. Separation papers

_____ 57. Service agreements and warranties

_____ 58. Social Security card

_____ 59. Social Security card belonging to spouse

_____ 60. Spouse's documents

_____ 61. Stock certificates not in brokerage or IRA account

_____ 62. Storage agreements

_____ 63. Titles (other than real property deeds or automobile titles)

_____ 64. Trust agreements

_____ 65. Valuables/collections (inventories, appraisals)

_____ 66. Veterans Administration papers

_____ 67. Visa, alien registration, and immigration status

_____ 68. Welfare or SSI status

DOCUMENT COLLECTION FORM

1. Adoption papers

Identify adoption agency and state.

Dates _____

Original or copy? (If a copy, note who has the original.) _____

Notes _____

_____

2. Annuity policies

Get copies of most recent statements.

Dates _____

Original or copy? (If a copy, note who has the original.) _____

Notes _____

_____

3. Automobile titles or leases

Auto insurance policies should show who has a lien on the title.

Dates _____

Original or copy? (If a copy, note who has the original.) _____

Notes _____

_____

4. Balance statements (checking, savings, Christmas Club, IRA, 401(k), 403(b), Keogh, credit union, money market, lines of credit, and so on)

List any authorized signers for automatic deposits, payments, and loans.

Dates _____

Original or copy? (If a copy, note who has the original.) _____

Notes _____

_____

5. Baptism records

Dates _____

Original or copy? (If a copy, note who has the original.) _____

Notes _____

_____

6. Bar/Bat Mitzvah records

Dates _____

Original or copy? (If a copy, note who has the original.) _____

Notes _____

_____

7. Birth certificate

Get multiple, state-certified copies.

Dates _____

Original or copy? (If a copy, note who has the original.) _____

Notes _____

_____

8. Bonds (not held in brokerage account)

If bearer bonds, are mature coupons attached? Write payment dates in the *Vital Information Form* (pages 9–33).

Dates _____

Original or copy? (If a copy, note who has the original.) _____

Notes _____

_____

9. Brokerage statements (stocks, bonds, mutual funds, and so on)

Who can initiate trades? Are margin loans permitted?

Dates_____

Original or copy? (If a copy, note who has the original.) _____

Notes _____

_____

10. Citizenship/naturalization papers

Include place of origin, date of entry, and initial visa status.

Dates_____

Original or copy? (If a copy, note who has the original.) _____

Notes _____

_____

11. Credit/debit cards

List issuers, account numbers, and expiration dates. Be sure to cancel unused cards to save fees.

Dates_____

Original or copy? (If a copy, note who has the original.) _____

Notes _____

_____

12. Death certificate of spouse (or prior spouse)

Get multiple, state-certified copies. These may be necessary to claim certain rights and benefits.

Dates_____

Original or copy? (If a copy, note who has the original.) _____

Notes _____

_____

13. Deeds to real property

Collect condo/co-op documents, title insurance policies, and surveys.

Dates _____

Original or copy? (If a copy, note who has the original.) _____

Notes _____

_____

14. Deferred compensation agreements

Dates _____

Original or copy? (If a copy, note who has the original.) _____

Notes _____

_____

15. Divorce decree, settlement agreements, and court orders

Include alimony and/or property settlements.

Dates _____

Original or copy? (If a copy, note who has the original.) _____

Notes _____

_____

16. Driver's license

Keep a copy of the license, even if it has expired (it may still be used as photo ID). Write down the number and expiration date.

Dates _____

Original or copy? (If a copy, note who has the original.) _____

Notes _____

_____

17. Employment history

Give a detailed history of employers, dates, positions, and reasons for leaving.

Dates _____

Original or copy? (If a copy, note who has the original.) _____

Notes _____

_____

18. Funeral/cremation, prepaid funeral, cemetery plot, organ donation

Include funeral home preference, any irrevocable Medicaid trust documents, organ donation information, and burial or cremation instructions.

Dates _____

Original or copy? (If a copy, note who has the original.) _____

Notes _____

_____

19. Gift tax returns (federal and state)

Include all.

Dates _____

Original or copy? (If a copy, note who has the original.) _____

Notes _____

_____

20. Group health booklets and ID cards

Include Medigap or post-retirement coverages and prenotification criteria. Copy front and back of ID cards.

Dates _____

Original or copy? (If a copy, note who has the original.) _____

Notes _____

_____

21. Group life policies, certificates, booklets

Include accidental coverages.

Dates_____

Original or copy? (If a copy, note who has the original.)_____

Notes_____

_____

22. Income tax returns (federal, state, and local) for the last seven years

Collect schedules, evidence of payment (or exemption from filing or paying), and information on any open audits.

Dates_____

Original or copy? (If a copy, note who has the original.)_____

Notes_____

_____

23. Inheritance documents

Note whether the elderly person has received everything he or she has inherited.

Dates_____

Original or copy? (If a copy, note who has the original.)_____

Notes_____

_____

24. Inventory of possessions in the home

Can be a detailed list or a videotape. Keep this with the *Vital Information Form* (pages 9–33).

Dates_____

Original or copy? (If a copy, note who has the original.)_____

Notes_____

_____

25. Investment club agreement

Include any obligation to make contributions, as well as the process for getting out of the agreement.

Dates _____

Original or copy? (If a copy, note who has the original.) _____

Notes _____

_____

26. Last will and testament, including codicils

Dates _____

Original or copy? (If a copy, note who has the original.) _____

Notes _____

_____

27. Legal claims as plaintiff, defendant, or class member

A class member may have a right to money claimed in a class-action lawsuit. Make sure the lawyer has all the necessary facts and documents.

Dates _____

Original or copy? (If a copy, note who has the original.) _____

Notes _____

_____

28. Life insurance policies, certificates of insurance

Policies will usually be term or whole life. Is there any cash value to these policies? Are there any outstanding loans?

Dates _____

Original or copy? (If a copy, note who has the original.) _____

Notes _____

_____

29. Living will

Does it meet state requirements? Who has a copy? Has an agent been appointed?

Dates _____

Original or copy? (If a copy, note who has the original.) _____

Notes_____

_____

30. Loans or debts due to the elderly person

Get copies of notes or written obligations. If a verbal promise was made to pay back the money, try to get it in writing.

Dates _____

Original or copy? (If a copy, note who has the original.) _____

Notes_____

_____

31. Loans or debts owed by the elderly person

Get copies of notes or written obligations.

Dates _____

Original or copy? (If a copy, note who has the original.) _____

Notes_____

_____

32. Long-term care insurance policy, booklet

What benefits is the person entitled to? Has he or she applied for these benefits? If benefits are being paid, find out how much longer they'll be paid.

Dates _____

Original or copy? (If a copy, note who has the original.) _____

Notes_____

_____

33. Marriage certificate

Make sure it has been certified by the appropriate governmental body.

Dates_____

Original or copy? (If a copy, note who has the original.) _____

Notes _____

_____

34. Medicaid beneficiary ID

Include ID number and a letter from Medicaid confirming eligibility. If eligibility is pending, give the status, a calculation of assets owned, a list of assets transferred, and the eligibility status of spouse.

Dates_____

Original or copy? (If a copy, note who has the original.) _____

Notes _____

_____

35. Medicare ID

Determine current year deductible, co-pay status, and how many of the 100 long-term care days have been used.

Dates_____

Original or copy? (If a copy, note who has the original.) _____

Notes _____

_____

36. Membership list

List all clubs, associations, and societies the person belongs to. What are the membership benefits, dues, and minimum payments?

Dates_____

Original or copy? (If a copy, note who has the original.) _____

Notes _____

_____

37. Military discharge certificate

Include military ID number.

Dates _____

Original or copy? (If a copy, note who has the original.) _____

Notes _____

_____

38. Mortgages for each property

Include reverse mortgages and home equity loans secured by second mortgages.

Dates _____

Original or copy? (If a copy, note who has the original.) _____

Notes _____

_____

39. Mortgage insurance

Is mortgage insurance still needed? Will term insurance cover the payoff amount?

Dates _____

Original or copy? (If a copy, note who has the original.) _____

Notes _____

_____

40. Organ donor card

Does it meet state requirements? Give a copy of this card to your local organ procurement agency, and attach a copy to the durable healthcare power of attorney.

Dates _____

Original or copy? (If a copy, note who has the original.) _____

Notes _____

_____

41. Partnerships (general and limited)

Collect partnership documents and any buy/sell agreements.

Dates _____

Original or copy? (If a copy, note who has the original.) _____

Notes _____

_____

42. Passport

Write down the number and expiration date, and get a copy of the identification page of the passport.

Dates _____

Original or copy? (If a copy, note who has the original.) _____

Notes _____

_____

43. Pension or retirement plans (booklets, statements, benefit summaries, retiree health)

Are any benefits or survivorship benefits payable?

Dates _____

Original or copy? (If a copy, note who has the original.) _____

Notes _____

_____

44. Personal address book

Use this to create a contact list of family and friends. (See page 223.)

Dates _____

Original or copy? (If a copy, note who has the original.) _____

Notes _____

_____

45. Personal contracts

Collect all current contracts (CCRC, home care agency, and so on).

Dates _____

Original or copy? (If a copy, note who has the original.) _____

Notes _____

_____

46. Pet information

Include information about vaccinations, pet sitters, the animal hospital or vet, medications, and burial plans.

Dates _____

Original or copy? (If a copy, note who has the original.) _____

Notes _____

_____

47. Powers of attorney (durable healthcare)

Does it meet state requirements? List the agent's name, address, and phone number. Who has copies of the power of attorney?

Dates _____

Original or copy? (If a copy, note who has the original.) _____

Notes _____

_____

48. Powers of attorney (general or special)

Summarize the powers granted and list the agent's name, address, and phone number. Who has copies of the power of attorney? Is it durable?

Dates _____

Original or copy? (If a copy, note who has the original.) _____

Notes _____

_____

49. Prenuptial or postnuptial agreement

Dates _____

Original or copy? (If a copy, note who has the original.) _____

Notes _____

_____

50. Prescription drug plans (ID cards, booklet)

Determine co-pay and deductible status. Collect medication records as well as mail-order pharmacy information.

Dates _____

Original or copy? (If a copy, note who has the original.) _____

Notes _____

_____

51. Property and casualty insurance

Dates _____

Original or copy? (If a copy, note who has the original.) _____

Notes _____

_____

52. Property and school tax receipts from the past three years.

Dates _____

Original or copy? (If a copy, note who has the original.) _____

Notes _____

_____

53. Rental/time share agreements

Include leases, agreement dates, and other commitments, whether the person is the lessor or lessee.

Dates _____

Original or copy? (If a copy, note who has the original.) _____

Notes _____

_____

54. Safety deposit box and home safe contents

List the contents stored in the box/safe, and note the location. Also note the location of the key or combination.

Dates _____

Original or copy? (If a copy, note who has the original.) _____

Notes _____

_____

55. Savings bonds

List maturity dates.

Dates _____

Original or copy? (If a copy, note who has the original.) _____

Notes _____

_____

56. Separation papers

Are there any support agreements?

Dates _____

Original or copy? (If a copy, note who has the original.) _____

Notes _____

_____

57. Service agreements and warranties

Collect those that are still valid. List major appliances and expiration dates.

Dates _____

Original or copy? (If a copy, note who has the original.) _____

Notes _____

_____

58. Social Security card

Get a copy of the card and the entitlement statement from the Social Security Administration. Are there forty quarters of earnings? Is the money automatically deposited into a bank account?

Dates _____

Original or copy? (If a copy, note who has the original.) _____

Notes _____

_____

59. Social Security card belonging to spouse

Get a copy of the card and the entitlement statement from the Social Security Administration. Are there forty quarters of earnings? Is the money automatically deposited into a bank account?

Dates _____

Original or copy? (If a copy, note who has the original.) _____

Notes _____

_____

60. Spouse's documents

Include important documents that could create obligations or affect benefits, including employment history and personally owned assets.

Dates _____

Original or copy? (If a copy, note who has the original.) _____

Notes _____

_____

61. Stock certificates not in brokerage or IRA account

Determine how stock is held (individually or jointly).

Dates _____

Original or copy? (If a copy, note who has the original.) _____

Notes _____

_____

62. Storage agreements

List locations, items in storage, and where the keys are.

Dates _____

Original or copy? (If a copy, note who has the original.) _____

Notes _____

_____

63. Titles (other than real property deeds or automobile titles)

Include titles to boats and stadium seats.

Dates _____

Original or copy? (If a copy, note who has the original.) _____

Notes _____

_____

64. Trust agreements

These are generally estate planning documents.

Dates _____

Original or copy? (If a copy, note who has the original.) _____

Notes _____

_____

65. Valuables/collections (inventories, appraisals)

Are inventories and appraisals up-to-date?

Dates _____

Original or copy? (If a copy, note who has the original.) _____

Notes _____

_____

66. Veterans Administration papers

Collect applications, proof of eligibility, discharge papers, and burial requests.

Dates _____

Original or copy? (If a copy, note who has the original.) _____

Notes _____

_____

67. Visa, alien registration, and immigration status

If the elderly person is not a citizen, collect immigration documents and proof of his or her entitlement to benefits.

Dates _____

Original or copy? (If a copy, note who has the original.) _____

Notes _____

_____

68. Welfare or SSI status

Collect documents that show entitlement to welfare, food stamps, SSI, or other government benefits.

Dates _____

Original or copy? (If a copy, note who has the original.) _____

Notes _____

_____

Telephone Contact Lists

This section includes the following contact lists:
- *Emergency Contacts*
- *Caregiver's Emergency Contacts*
- *General Contact List*
- *Caregiver Information*
- *Networking and References List*
- *Family and Friends List*
- *Volunteers List*

Emergency Contacts contains telephone numbers for an elderly person to use in an emergency. Keep a copy of this list near every telephone in the elderly person's home, and make a copy for him or her to carry in a purse or wallet (along with the *Medication Summary, Basic Medical Information,* and *Medical History*). As the caregiver, you should have a copy of this list as well.

Caregiver's Emergency Contacts contains emergency information for the caregiver. It does not duplicate the elderly person's emergency contact list, because the people you would need to contact in an emergency may be very different from those the elderly person would contact. Keep this list with you at all times. If you're a long-distance caregiver, you should also have phone books from the elderly person's community. When you're not sure whom to call, it's easier to page through a telephone book than try to arrange help through directory assistance.

The *General Contact List* is a fairly comprehensive list for both the elderly person and the caregiver. While it contains many numbers you may never use, it provides a handy reference when you need it. Both of you should keep a copy in your home.

The *Caregiver Information* form is especially important for long-distance caregivers. A copy should be given to the elderly person's physician,

clergy, friends, home healthcare aides, neighbors, and anyone else who may need to contact you in an emergency. You may want to attach a $5 pre-paid phone card to emphasize how important it is for them to call you at any time.

As you network, search for references, and specific goods or services on behalf of the elderly person, and record your contacts on the *Networking and References List*. Write down each person or organization you contact, the date, telephone number, person you spoke with, purpose of the call, and comments that may be helpful if you need to contact the person later.

Together, you and the elderly person can fill out the *Family and Friends List* using the elderly person's personal address book. This list should include all the friends and family members that the elderly person wants you to contact in the event of an emergency or death. It should also note which family members are blood relatives.

The *Volunteers List* is a list of neighbors, friends, church members, and family who have volunteered to help the elderly person in some way. They may have offered their time, money, or special expertise. When people volunteer to help, take them up on it. Use this list to record their names, telephone numbers, what they have volunteered to do, and when or how often they will do it. If you are a long-distance caregiver, take advantage of your visits to the elderly person by trying to add to this list and arrange for backups in case a volunteer goes on vacation, gets sick, or cancels unexpectedly. Depending on the importance of the service, you may wish to periodically acknowledge each volunteer's kindness with a note or small gift.

EMERGENCY CONTACTS

Write this list in heavy black ink, and make sure it's large enough so the elderly person can read it without his or her glasses. Place a copy by every telephone in the home, and encourage the elderly person to carry a copy whenever he or she leaves home. If the elderly person lives in an area where 911 calls the police, fire department, and emergency rescue, enter 911 in the first three lines. Feel free to add to this list as you see fit.

	Name	Telephone number
Police		
Fire		
Emergency rescue		
Doctor 1 (office)		
Doctor 1 (pager)		
Doctor 2 (office)		
Doctor 2 (pager)		
Caregiver (primary)		
Pharmacy		
Dentist		
Home healthcare agency		
Visiting nurse		
Home healthcare aide		
Therapist 1 (in-home)		

Therapist 2 (in-home) _____ _____

Medical supply company _____ _____

Assistive device supplier _____ _____

Social worker _____ _____

Close family member _____ _____

Neighbor 1 _____ _____

Neighbor 2 _____ _____

Friend 1 _____ _____

Friend 2 _____ _____

Clergy _____ _____

Insurance agent _____ _____

Lawyer _____ _____

_____ _____ _____

_____ _____ _____

_____ _____ _____

_____ _____ _____

_____ _____ _____

CAREGIVER EMERGENCY CONTACTS

In any crisis, you need to consider what to do about home or pet care. In addition, you may need to contact in-home service providers and stop the mail and newspaper deliveries.

	Name	Telephone number	Comments
Geriatric care manager			
Primary care doctor			
Hospital			
Hospital discharge planner			
Home healthcare agency			
Nursing service			
Neighbor 1			
Neighbor 2			
House sitter			
Pet sitter			
Area Agency on Aging			
Newspaper			Stop paper
Post office			Stop mail
Travel agent			
Airline			
Car rental company			
Hotel (or place you'll be staying)			

GENERAL CONTACT LIST

	Name	Address	Telephone number
Accountant			
Air conditioner repair			
Animal hospital			
Appliance repair			
Area Agency on Aging			
Banker			
Beautician/barber			
Bookkeeper			
Broker			
Cable/satellite provider			
Carpenter			
Church/synagogue/mosque			
Clergy			
Dentist			
Doctor 1 (billing)			
Doctor 1 (office)			
Doctor 2 (billing)			
Doctor 2 (office)			
Elderlaw attorney			
Electric company			
Electrician			
Estate lawyer			
Eye doctor			
Eyeglasses supplier			
Financial planner			
Furnace			
Gas company			
Geriatric care manager			

Handyman	_____	_____	_____
Health insurance agent	_____	_____	_____
Health insurance company	_____	_____	_____
Health insurance (precertification)	_____	_____	_____
Healthcare aide 1	_____	_____	_____
Healthcare aide 2	_____	_____	_____
Hearing care	_____	_____	_____
Home care aide	_____	_____	_____
Home healthcare agency	_____	_____	_____
Home security company (know code and password)	_____	_____	_____
Hospital (billing)	_____	_____	_____
Hospital (general)	_____	_____	_____
Hospital discharge planner	_____	_____	_____
House sitter	_____	_____	_____
Insurance agent: automobile	_____	_____	_____
Insurance agent: homeowners	_____	_____	_____
Insurance agent: other	_____	_____	_____
Landlord	_____	_____	_____
Legal guardian	_____	_____	_____
Locksmith	_____	_____	_____
Meals-on-Wheels	_____	_____	_____
Medical supplies 1	_____	_____	_____
Medical supplies 2	_____	_____	_____
Newspaper 1	_____	_____	_____
Newspaper 2	_____	_____	_____
Oil delivery company	_____	_____	_____

Pet sitter _____ _____ _____

Pharmacy (local) _____ _____ _____

Pharmacy (mail-in) _____ _____ _____

Plumber _____ _____ _____

Podiatrist _____ _____ _____

Property manager _____ _____ _____

Property security _____ _____ _____

Senior center _____ _____ _____

Snow removal _____ _____ _____

Social worker _____ _____ _____

Storage/locker _____ _____ _____

Tax preparer _____ _____ _____

Telephone repair _____ _____ _____

Therapist 1 (in-home) _____ _____ _____

Therapist 2 (in-home) _____ _____ _____

Therapy office 1 _____ _____ _____

Therapy office 2 _____ _____ _____

Veterinarian _____ _____ _____

Visiting nurse 1 _____ _____ _____

Visiting nurse 2 _____ _____ _____

Visiting nurse 3 _____ _____ _____

Yard/landscape service _____ _____ _____

_____ _____ _____ _____

_____ _____ _____ _____

_____ _____ _____ _____

_____ _____ _____ _____

_____ _____ _____ _____

_____ _____ _____ _____

A Family Caregiver's Guide to Planning and Decision Making for the Elderly © 1999 James A. Wilkinson

CAREGIVER INFORMATION

I am a caregiver for _____. I would like to be called if any emergency develops, if you see anything unusual, or if you get the feeling that everything is not okay. Because I cannot be there as much as I would like, it is very important that others tell me what they see and hear.

_____

(name)

_____

(name of my spouse or other relative)

I can be reached at:

(work telephone number) _____

(home telephone number) _____

(spouse/relative work telephone number) _____

(spouse/relative home telephone number) _____

I am normally at home after _____. If I am not at home during the day and it is not an emergency, please leave a message and I will call you back. If it is an emergency, please call my work number or that of my spouse/relative. If he or she cannot be reached, please contact:

_____

(name)

_____

(relationship to elderly person)

(work telephone number) _____

(home telephone number) _____

NETWORKING AND REFERENCES LIST

This list can be helpful when you are checking references or networking on behalf of the elderly person. You may want to make several copies of this list. Record the name and phone number of each person you call, the date and purpose of the call, and his or her responses to your questions.

Person/agency called _____ Date _____

Phone number _____

Person you spoke to _____

Purpose of call _____

Comments _____

_____

_____

Person/agency called _____ Date _____

Phone number _____

Person you spoke to _____

Purpose of call _____

Comments _____

_____

_____

Person/agency called _____ Date _____

Phone number _____

Person you spoke to _____

Purpose of call _____

Comments _____

_____

_____

FAMILY AND FRIENDS LIST

Most of the information on this list can be taken from the elderly person's personal address book. You may want to make several copies of this list. Write down the elderly person's friends and family members whom you may need to contact if the person's condition changes. You can make notes about when to call each person, in what priority, and so forth.

Name_____

Address _____

Telephone number _____

Blood relative? _____

Notes_____

_____

_____

Name_____

Address _____

Telephone number _____

Blood relative? _____

Notes_____

_____

_____

Name_____

Address _____

Telephone number _____

Blood relative? _____

Notes_____

_____

_____

VOLUNTEERS LIST

This list records information about individuals who have volunteered to help the elderly person. You may want to make several copies of this list. Any time someone offers their assistance, take down his or her information. Even if you don't need help today, you may have to call on this person in the future.

Name_____

Service offered _____

When and how often_____

Telephone number _____

Name_____

Service offered _____

When and how often_____

Telephone number _____

Name_____

Service offered _____

When and how often_____

Telephone number _____

Name_____

Service offered _____

When and how often_____

Telephone number _____

Name_____

Service offered _____

When and how often_____

Telephone number _____

Other Sources of Information

Organization and Hotlines

The organizations and hotlines that follow will help the elderly and their caregivers find additional information about health, eldercare services, aging, financial planning, and so forth.

Please note that many resources may also have an Internet address listed in Internet Sites beginning on page 255. All addresses and numbers are subject to change.

Abuse and Neglect

National Center on Elder Abuse
810 First Street N.E., Suite 500
Washington, DC 20002
(202) 682-2470

National Organization for Victim Assistance
1757 Park Road N.W.
Washington, DC 20010
(202) 232-6682
Fax (202) 462-2255

African-American Services

Black Elderly Legal Assistance
Support Project
National Bar Association
1225 11th Street N.W.
Washington, DC 20001
(202) 842-3900

National Caucus and Center on
the Black Aged
1424 K Street N.W., Suite 500
Washington, DC 20005
(202) 637-8400

Alcohol and Drugs

National Clearinghouse for Alcohol and
Drug Information
P.O. Box 2345
Rockville, MD 20825-2345
1-800-729-6686

National Council on Alcoholism and Drug
Dependence
12 W. 21st Street, Seventh Floor
New York, NY 10010
(212) 206-6770
1-800-622-2255
Fax (212) 645-1690

Alzheimer's Disease

Alzheimer's Association
919 N. Michigan Avenue, Suite 1000
Chicago, IL 60611
(312) 335-8700
1-800-272-3900
Fax (312) 335-8882

Alzheimer's Disease Education
and Referral Center
P.O. Box 8250
Silver Springs, MD 20907-8250
(301) 495-3311
1-800-438-4380
Fax (301) 495-3334

Alzheimer's Family Relief Program
American Health Assistance Foundation
15825 Shady Grove Road, Suite 140
Rockville, MD 20850
1-800-437-AHAF (437-2423)

Arthritis

Arthritis Foundation
P.O. Box 6065
Daytona Beach, FL 32122
(904) 258-1170
1-800-282-9487

National Arthritis, Musculoskeletal & Skin
Diseases Information Clearinghouse
1 AMS Circle
Bethesda, MD 20892-3675
(301) 495-4484

Asian Services

Japanese-American Citizens League
1765 Sutter Street
San Francisco, CA 94115
(415) 921-5225

National Asian Pacific Center on Aging
Melbourne Tower
1511 Third Avenue, Suite 914
Seattle, WA 98101-1626
(206) 624-1221

Organization of Chinese Americans
1001 Connecticut Avenue N.W., Room 707
Washington, DC 20036
(202) 223-5500
Fax (202) 296-0540

Cancer

American Cancer Society
1599 Clifton Road N.E.
Atlanta, GA 30329
(404) 320-3333
1-800-ACS-2345 (227-2345)

Make Today Count, Inc.
Mid-American Cancer Center
1235 E. Cherokee Street
Springfield, MO 65804
1-800-432-2273

National Cancer Institute
Cancer Information Service (CIS)
1-800-4-CANCER

National Coalition for Cancer Survivorship
1010 Wayne Avenue, Suite 505
Silver Spring, MD 20910
1-888-650-9127

The Skin Cancer Foundation
245 Fifth Avenue, Suite 2402
New York, NY 10016
(212) 725-5176
1-800-SKIN-490 (754-6490)
Fax (212) 725-5751

Chronic Pain

American Chronic Pain Association
P.O. Box 850
Rocklin, CA 95677
(916) 632-0922

Dentistry

American Dental Association
211 E. Chicago Avenue
Chicago, IL 60611-2678
(312) 440-2593

National Institute of Dental Research
Information Office
Building 31, Room 5B-49
31 Center Drive MSC 2190
Bethesda, MD 20892-2190
(301) 496-4261

Diabetes

American Diabetes Association
1660 Duke Street
Alexandria, VA 22314
(703) 549-1500
1-800-DIABETES (342-2383)

National Diabetes Information
Clearinghouse
One Information Way
Bethesda, MD 20892-3560
(301) 654-3327

National Institute of Diabetes and
Digestive and Kidney Diseases
Information Office
Building 31, Room 9A-04
31 Center Drive MSC 2560
Bethesda, MD 20892-2560
(301) 496-3583

Digestive Disorders

National Digestive Diseases
Information Clearinghouse
Two Information Way
Bethesda, MD 20892-3570
(301) 654-3810

National Institute of Diabetes and
Digestive and Kidney Diseases
Information Office
Building 31, Room 9A-04
31 Center Drive MSC 2560
Bethesda, MD 20892-2560
(301) 496-3583

Financial Services

American Institute of Certified
Public Accountants
Financial Management
Harborside Financial Center
201 Plaza Three
Jersey City, NJ 07311-3881
1-800-862-4272

Institute of Certified Financial Planners
3801 E. Florida Avenue, Suite 708
Denver, CO 80210
(303) 759-4900
1-800-282-7526

International Association for
Financial Planning
5775 Glenridge Drive N.E., Suite B-300
Atlanta, GA 30328
1-800-945-4237
Fax (404) 845-3660

National Association of Personal
Financial Advisors
355 W. Dundee Road, Suite 200
Buffalo Grove, IL 60089
(847) 537-7722
1-800-366-2732

Fitness and Nutrition

Aging Well
Exercises for Seniors
128 Oakwood Avenue
Pittsburgh, PA 15229
(412) 931-5117

American Dietetic Association
216 W. Jackson Boulevard
Chicago, IL 60606-6995
(312) 899-0040
1-800-877-1600 (Publications Service)
1-800-366-1655 (Consumer Nutrition)

National Senior Sports Association
83 Princeton Avenue
Hopewell, NJ 08525
(609) 466-0022
1-800-752-9718
Fax (609) 466-9366

Foot Care

American Podiatric Medical Association
9312 Old Georgetown Road
Bethesda, MD 20814
(301) 571-9200
1-800-FOOT-CARE (366-8227)
Fax (301) 530-2752

Funeral and Cemetery Information

Cemetery Consumer Service Council
P.O. Box 2028
Reston, VA 20195-0028
(703) 391-8407

Funeral Service Consumer Assistance
Program
P.O. Box 486
Elm Grove, WI 53122-0486
1-800-662-7666

Service Corporation International
1929 Allen Parkway
Houston, TX 77019
1-800-9-CARING (922-7464)

General Information for Caregivers

Administration on Aging
Department of Health and Human Services
330 Independence Avenue S.W.
Washington, DC 20201
(202) 619-0724
1-800-677-1116 (eldercare locator)
Fax (202) 401-7620

Aging Network Services
4400 East-West Highway, Suite 907
Bethesda, MD 20814
(301) 657-4329

Aging with Dignity
P.O. Box 1661
Tallahassee, FL 32302-1661
1-800-562-1931

American Association of Homes
and Services for the Aging
901 E Street N.W., Suite 500
Washington, DC 20004-2037
(202) 783-2242
1-800-508-9442

Children of Aging Parents
1609 Woodburne Road, Suite 302A
Levittown, PA 19057
(215) 945-6900
1-800-227-7294
Fax (215) 945-8720

Christmas in April
4614 Wisconsin Avenue N.W.
Washington, DC 20016
(202) 362-1611
Fax (202) 244-9551

Consumer Information Center
P.O. Box WWW
Pueblo, CO 81009
1-888-878-3256

Council of Better Business Bureaus, Inc.
4200 Wilson Boulevard, Suite 800
Arlington, VA 22203
(703) 276-0100
Fax (703) 525-8277

Eldercare Locator
1-800-677-1116

Family Resource Service
1400 Union Meeting Road, Suite 102
Blue Bell, PA 19422
1-800-847-5437

Federal Trade Commission
Office of Public Affairs
6th Street and Pennsylvania Avenue N.W.
Room 421
Washington, DC 20580
(202) 382-4357 (to locate office near you)

Joint Commission on Accreditation of
Healthcare Organizations
One Renaissance Boulevard
Oak Brook Terrace, IL 60181
(630) 792-5000

National Association of Area Agencies
on Aging
1112 16th Street N.W., Suite 100
Washington, DC 20036-4823
(202) 296-8130
Fax (202) 296-8134

National Consumers League
1701 K Street N.W., Suite 1200
Washington, DC 20006
(202) 835-3323
Fax (202) 835-0747

National Fraud Information Center
1-800-876-7060

National Family Caregivers Association
10605 Concord Street, Suite 501
Kensington, MD 20895-2504
1-800-896-3650

Shepherd's Centers of America
W. Armor Boulevard, Suite 201
Kansas City, MO 64131
(816) 960-2022
Fax (816) 960-1083

General Information for the Elderly

American Association of Retired Persons
(AARP)
601 E. Street N.W.
Washington, DC 20049
1-800-424-3410
Fax (202) 434-7681

American Geriatrics Society
770 Lexington Avenue, Suite 300
New York, NY 10021
(212) 308-1414
Fax (212) 832-8646

American Society on Aging
833 Market Street, Suite 511
San Francisco, CA 94103
(415) 974-9600
1-800-537-9728
Fax (415) 974-0300

Center for the Study of Aging
1331 H Street N.W.
Washington, DC 20005
(202) 737-4650
1-800-221-4272
Fax (202) 783-1931

Elderhostel
75 Federal Street
Boston, MA 02110-1941
(617) 426-7788

Grandparent Information Center
601 E Street N.W.
Washington, DC 20049
(202) 434-2296

Gray Panthers
2025 Pennsylvania Avenue N.W., Suite 821
Washington, DC 20006
(202) 466-3132
1-800-280-5362
Fax (202) 466-3133

Grief Recovery Institute
8306 Wilshire Boulevard, Suite 21A
Beverly Hills, CA 90211
(213) 650-1234
1-800-445-4808

National Aging Information Center
330 Independence Avenue S.W., Room 4656
Washington, DC 20201
(202) 619-7501

National Council on the Aging
409 Third Street S.W., Suite 200
Washington, DC 20024
(202) 479-1200
1-800-424-9046
Fax (202) 479-0735

National Council of Senior Citizens
8403 Colesville Road, Suite 1200
Silver Springs, MD 20910
(301) 578-8800
Fax (301) 578-8999

National Institute on Aging
Public Information Office
Building 31, Room 5C27
31 Center Drive MSC 2292
Bethesda, MD 20892-2292
1-800-222-2225

Older Adult Service and Information System
(OASIS)
7710 Carondelet Avenue, Suite 125
St. Louis, MO 63105
(314) 862-2933
Fax (314) 862-2149

United Way of America
701 N. Fairfax Street
Alexandria, VA 22314-2045
(703) 836-7100
Fax (703) 683-7813

Well Spouse Foundation
610 Lexington Avenue, Suite 208
New York, NY 10022
(212) 644-1241
Fax (212) 644-1338

Widowed Persons Service
601 E Street N.W.
Washington, DC 20049
(202) 434-2260
Fax (202) 434-6474

Health and Medicine

American Academy of Orthopedic Surgeons
6300 N. River Road
Rosemont, IL 60018-4262
(708) 384-4257
1-800-787-4366

American Academy of Physical Medicine
and Rehabilitation
One IBM Plaza, Suite 2500
Chicago, IL 60611
(312) 464-9700
Fax (312) 464-0227

American Medical Association
515 N. State Street
Chicago, IL 60610
(312) 464-5000
Fax (312) 464-4184

American Nurses Association
600 Maryland Avenue S.W., Suite 100W
Washington, DC 20024-2571
(202) 554-4444
1-800-274-4262
Fax (202) 651-7001

American Occupational Therapy Association
4720 Montgomery Lane
P.O. Box 31220
Bethesda, MD 20824-1220
(301) 652-2682
Fax (301) 652-7711

American Pharmaceutical Association
2215 Constitution Avenue N.W.
Washington, DC 20037
(202) 628-4410
1-800-237-2742
Fax (202) 783-2351

American Physical Therapy Association
1111 N. Fairfax Street
Alexandria, VA 22314
(703) 684-2782

American Red Cross
430 17th Street N.W.
Washington, DC 20006
(202) 728-6400

American Trauma Society
8903 Presidential Parkway, Suite 512
Upper Marlboro, MD 20772
(301) 420-4189
1-800-556-7890
Fax (301) 420-0617

Center for the Study of Pharmacy and
Therapeutics for the Elderly
School of Pharmacy
University of Maryland at Baltimore
20 N. Pine Street
Baltimore, MD 21201-1180
(410) 706-3011
Fax (410) 706-0897

National Council on Patient Information
and Education
666 11th Street N.W., Suite 810
Washington, DC 20001
(202) 347-6711
Fax (202) 638-0773

National Health Council
1730 M Street N.W., Suite 500
Washington, DC 20036
(202) 785-3910
Fax (202) 785-5923

National Health Information Center Hotline
U.S. Department of Health and Human
Services
1-800-336-4797

National Institute of Health
9000 Rockville Pike
Bethesda, MD 20892
(301) 496-3583
Fax (301) 496-7422

National League for Nursing (NLN)
61 Broadway, 33rd Floor
New York, NY 10006
1-800-669-1656

National Rehabilitation Information Center
8455 Colesville Road, Suite 935
Silver Spring, MD 20910-3319
(301) 588-9284
1-800-346-2742

Visiting Nurses Association of America
11 Deacon Street, Suite 910
Boston, MA 02108
1-800-426-2547
1-888-866-8773

Hearing Loss
American Speech-Language-Hearing
Foundation
10801 Rockville Pike
Rockville, MD 20852
(301) 897-7341

Better Hearing Institute
P.O. Box 1840
Washington, DC 20013
(703) 642-0580
1-800-EAR-WELL (327-9355)

Hearing Aid Helpline
16880 Middlebelt Road, Suite Four
Livonia, MI 48154
1-800-521-5247

National Information Center on Deafness
Gallaudet University
800 Florida Avenue N.E.
Washington, DC 20002-3695
(202) 651-5051
Fax (202) 651-5054

National Institute on Deafness & Other
Communication Disorders Clearinghouse
Information Office
Building 31, Room 3C-35
31 Center Drive MSC 2320
Bethesda, MD 20892-2320
(301) 496-7243

Self-Help for Hard of Hearing People, Inc.
7910 Woodmont Avenue, Suite 1200
Bethesda, MD 20814
(301) 657-2248
Fax (301) 913-9413

Vestibular Disorders Association
P.O. Box 4467
Portland, OR 97208-4467
(503) 229-7705

Heart Conditions
American Heart Association
7272 Greenville Avenue
Dallas, TX 75231
(214) 373-6300
1-800-242-8721

National Heart, Lung, and Blood Institute
Education Programs Information Center
P.O. Box 30105
Bethesda, MD 20824
(301) 251-1222
Fax (301) 251-1223

Hispanic Services

Meeting the Special Concerns of
Hispanic Older Women
National Hispanic Council on Aging
2713 Ontario Road N.W.
Washington, DC 20009
(202) 265-1288
Fax (202) 745-2522

National Association for Hispanic Elderly
1452 W. Temple Street, Suite 100
Los Angeles, CA 90026-1724
(213) 487-1922

National Hispanic Council on Aging
2713 Ontario Road N.W.
Washington, DC 20009
(202) 265-1288

Project Aliento
National Association for Hispanic Elderly
Asociacion Nacional Pro Personas Mayores
1452 W. Temple Street, Suite 100
Los Angeles, CA 90026-1724
(213) 487-1922
Fax (213) 202-5905

HIV/AIDS

HIV/AIDS Treatment Information Service
P.O. Box 6303
Rockville, MD 20849-6303
1-800-448-0440
Fax (301) 738-6616

Home Care

Meals-on-Wheels Association of America
1414 Prince Street, Suite 202
Alexandria, VA 22314
(703) 548-5558

National Adult Day Care Services Association
c/o National Council on the Aging
409 Third Street S.W., Suite 200
Washington, DC 20024
(202) 479-6682

National Association for Home Care
228 Seventh Street S.E.
Washington, DC 20003
(202) 547-7424

National Association of Professional
Geriatric Care Managers
1604 N. Country Club Road
Tucson, AZ 85716
(520) 881-8008

National Association of Social Workers
750 First Street N.E., Suite 700
Washington, DC 20002
(202) 408-8600
Fax (202) 336-8310

Hospice

Foundation for Hospice and Home Care
513 C Street N.E.
Washington, DC 20002
(202) 547-7424

Hospice Association of America
519 C Street N.E.
Washington, DC 20002
(202) 546-4759

Hospicelink
190 Westbrook Road
Essex, CT 06426
1-800-331-1620

National Hospice Organization
1901 N. Monroe Street, Suite 901
Arlington, VA 22209
(703) 243-5900
1-800-658-8898

Housing

American Healthcare Association
1201 L Street N.W.
Washington, DC 20005
(202) 842-4444
1-800-321-0343

Assisted Living Facility Association of
America
10300 Eaton Place, Suite 400
Fairfax, VA 22031
(703) 691-8100

National Citizens Coalition for
Nursing Home Reform
1424 16th Street N.W., Suite 202
Washington, DC 20036-2211
(202) 332-2275

National Resource and Policy Center on
Housing and Long-Term Care
University of Southern California
Andrus Gerontology Center
Los Angeles, CA 90089-0191
(213) 740-1364

National Shared Housing Resource Center
321 E. 25th Street
Baltimore, MD 21218
(410) 235-4454

Huntington's Disease

Huntington's Disease Society of America
158 W. 29th Street, Seventh Floor
New York, NY 10001-5300
(212) 242-1968
1-800-345-4372

Incontinence

National Association for Continence
P.O. Box 8310
Spartanburg, SC 29305-8310
(803) 579-7900
1-800-252-3337

The Simon Foundation for Continence
Box 815
Wilmette, IL 60091
(847) 864-3913
1-800-237-4666
Fax (847) 864-9758

Insurance

American Council of Life Insurance
1001 Pennsylvania Avenue N.W.
Washington, DC 20004-2599
(202) 624-2000

Health Insurance Association of America
555 13th Street N.W., Suite 600 East
Washington, DC 20004
(202) 824-1600

Insurance Information Institute
1730 Rhode Island Avenue N.W., Suite 710
Washington, DC 20036
(202) 833-1580

Medicare Hotline
1-800-638-6833

National Insurance Consumer Helpline
1-800-942-4242

Kidney and Urinary Care
American Urological Association
1120 N. Charles Street
Baltimore, MD 21201
(410) 727-1100
Fax (410) 468-1820

National Institute of Diabetes and Digestive
and Kidney Diseases Information Office
Building 31, Room 9A-04
31 Center Drive MSC 2560
Bethesda, MD 20892-2560
(301) 496-3583

National Kidney Foundation
30 E. 33rd Street
New York, NY 10016
(212) 889-2210
1-800-622-9010

National Kidney and Urologic Diseases
Information Clearinghouse
Three Information Way
Bethesda, MD 20892-3560
(301) 654-4415
Fax (301) 907-8906

Legal Services
American Bar Association Commission
on the Legal Problems of the Elderly
740 15th Street N.W.
Washington, DC 20005-1022
(202) 662-8690
Fax (202) 662-8698

Black Elderly Legal Assistance
Support Project
National Bar Association
1225 11th Street N.W.
Washington, DC 20001
(202) 842-3900

Choice in Dying, Inc.
1035 30th Street N.W.
Washington, DC 20007
1-800-989-9455

Legal Counsel for the Elderly (AARP)
601 E Street N.W.
Washington, DC 20049
(202) 434-2120

Legal Services for the Elderly
130 W. 42nd Street, 17th Floor
New York, NY 10036
(212) 391-0120
Fax (212) 719-1939

National Academy of Elderlaw Attorneys
1604 N. Country Club Road
Tucson, AZ 85716
(520) 881-4005

National Clearinghouse for Legal Services
205 W. Monroe, Second Floor
Chicago, IL 60606-5013
(312) 263-3830
Fax (312) 263-3846

National Legal Support for Elderly People
with Mental Disabilities
Judge David L. Bazelon Center for
Mental Health Law
1101 15th Street N.W., Suite 1212
Washington, DC 20005-5002
(202) 467-5730
Fax (202) 223-0409

National Senior Citizens Law Center
1101 14th Street N.W., Suite 400
Washington, DC 20005
(202) 289-6976
Fax (202) 289-7224

Leukemia

Leukemia Society of America
600 Third Avenue
New York, NY 10016
(212) 573-8484
1-800-955-4LSA (955-4572)
Fax (212) 856-9686

Lung Conditions

American Lung Association
1740 Broadway
New York, NY 10019-4374
(212) 315-8700
1-800-LUNG-USA (586-4872)
Fax (212) 265-5642

National Heart, Lung, and Blood Institute
Education Programs Information Center
P.O. Box 30105
Bethesda, MD 20824
(301) 251-1222
Fax (301) 251-1223

Lupus

Lupus Foundation of America
1300 Piccard Drive, Suite 200
Rockville, MD 20850-3226
(301) 670-9292
1-800-558-0121
1-800-558-0231 (Spanish)

Mental Health

American Association for Geriatric Psychiatry
7910 Woodmont Avenue, Suite 1350
Bethesda, MD 20814-3004
(301) 654-7850
Fax (301) 654-4137

American Psychiatric Association
1400 K Street N.W.
Washington, DC 20005
(202) 682-6325
Fax (202) 682-6255

American Psychological Association
P.O. Box 92984
Washington, DC 20002
(202) 336-5502
1-800-374-2721

National Institute of Mental Health
Information Resources and Inquiries Branch
5600 Fishers Lane, Room 7C-02
Rockville, MD 20857-8030
(301) 443-4513

National Mental Health Association
1021 Prince Street
Alexandria, VA 22314-2971
(703) 684-7722
1-800-969-6642
Fax (703) 684-5968

Multiple Sclerosis

National Multiple Sclerosis Society
733 Third Avenue, Sixth Floor
New York, NY 10017
(212) 986-3240
1-800-FIGHT MS (344-4867)

Native American Services

National Indian Council on Aging
10501 Montgomery Road N.E., Suite 210
Albuquerque, NM 87111-3846
(505) 292-2001

Native Elder Healthcare Resource Center
University of Colorado Health Sciences
Center
4455 E. 12th Avenue, Room 329
Colorado, CO 80220
(303) 315-9228
Fax (303) 315-9579

Osteoporosis

National Osteoporosis Foundation
1150 17th Street N.W., Suite 500
Washington, DC 20036-4603
(202) 223-2226
1-800-223-9994
Fax (202) 223-2237

Parkinson's Disease

American Parkinson's Disease Association
1250 Hylan Boulevard, Suite 4B
Staten Island, NY 10305
(718) 981-8001
1-800-223-2732
Fax (718) 981-4399

United Parkinson Foundation
833 W. Washington Boulevard
Chicago, IL 60607
(312) 733-1893
Fax (312) 664-2344

Pension

Pension Rights Center
918 16th Street N.W., Suite 704
Washington, DC 20006
(202) 296-3776

Religious Organizations

B'nai B'rith
1640 Rhode Island Avenue N.W.
Washington, DC 20036
(202) 857-6600
Fax (202) 857-1099

Catholic Charities USA
1731 King Street, Suite 200
Alexandria, VA 22314
(703) 549-1390

Elder Support Network
Association of Jewish Family
and Children's Agencies
1-800-634-7346

National Interfaith Coalition on Aging
National Council on the Aging
409 Third Street S.W., Suite 200
Washington, DC 20024
(202) 479-1200

National Jewish Medical and
Research Center
1400 Jackson Street
Denver, CO 80206
1-800-222-LUNG (5864)

Safety

Medic Alert Foundation
P.O. Box 381009
Turlock, CA 95382
(209) 668-3333
1-800-344-3226
Fax (209) 669-2450

National Safety Council
1121 Spring Lake Drive
Itasca, IL 60143-3201
(630) 285-1121
1-800-621-7619
Fax (630) 285-0797

Skin Conditions

National Arthritis, Musculoskeletal & Skin
Diseases Information Clearinghouse
One AMS Circle
Bethesda, MD 20892-3675
(301) 495-4484

National Psoriasis Foundation
6600 S.W. 92nd Avenue, Suite 300
Portland, OR 97223
(503) 244-7404
1-800-723-9166
Fax (503) 245-0626

Sleep Disorders

National Sleep Foundation
729 15th Street N.W., Fourth Floor
Washington, DC 20005
(202) 347-3471

Social Security

National Committee to Preserve
Social Security and Medicare
Ten G Street N.E., Suite 600
Washington, DC 20002
(202) 822-9459
1-800-998-0180

National Organization of Social Security
Claimants Representatives
Six Prospect Street
Midland Park, NJ 07432
(201) 444-1415
1-800-431-2804

Social Security Administration
Office of Public Inquiries
6401 Security Boulevard, Room 4J5
Baltimore, MD 21235
(410) 965-7700
1-800-772-1213

Stroke

National Institute of Neurological Disorders
and Stroke (NINDS)
Information Office
Building 31, Room 8A-O6
31 Center Drive MSC 2540
Bethesda, MD 20892-2540
(301) 496-5751
1-800-352-9424

National Stroke Association
96 Iverness Drive E., Suite One
Englewood, CO 80112-5112
(303) 649-9299
Fax (303) 649-1328
1-800-STROKES (787-6537)

Tinnitus

American Tinnitus Association
P.O. Box 5
Portland, OR 97207
(503) 248-9985
Fax (503) 248-0024

Veteran's Affairs

Civilian Health and Medical Program of the
Uniformed Services (CHAMPUS)
P.O. Box 65024
Denver, CO 80206-9024
1-800-733-8387 (claims processing)

U.S. Department of Veteran's Affairs
Office of Public Affairs
810 Vermont Avenue N.W.
Washington, DC 20420
1-800-827-1000
(benefits information and claims assistance)
1-800-669-8477 (life insurance)

Visual Problems

American Academy of Ophthalmology
665 Beach Street
San Francisco, CA 94109
(415) 561-8500

American Council of the Blind
1155 15th Street N.W., Suite 720
Washington, DC 20005
(202) 467-5081
1-800-424-8666
Fax (202) 467-5085

American Foundation for the Blind
11 Penn Plaza, Suite 300
New York, NY 10001
(212) 502-7600
1-800-232-5463
Fax (212) 502-7777

American Optometric Association
243 N. Lindbergh Boulevard
St. Louis, MO 63141
(314) 991-4100
Fax (314) 991-4101

Better Vision Institute
1655 N. Ft. Myer Drive, Suite 200
Rosslyn, VA 22209
(703) 243-1508
1-800-424-8422
Fax (703) 243-1537

National Association for Visually
Handicapped (NAVH)
Eastern States:
22 W. 21st Street, Sixth Floor
New York, NY 10010
(212) 889-3141

National Association for Visually
Handicapped (NAVH)
Western States:
3201 Balboa Street
San Francisco, CA 94121
(415) 221-3201

National Center for Vision and Aging
The Lighthouse, Inc.
111 E. 59th Street
New York, NY 10022
(212) 821-9200
1-800-334-5497
Fax (212) 821-9713

National Eyecare Project
1-800-222-EYES (3937)

National Eye Institute
Information Office
Building 31, Room 6A32
31 Center Drive MSC 2510
Bethesda, MD 20892-2510
(301) 496-5248
Fax (301) 402-1065

National Library Service for the Blind &
Physically Handicapped Hotline
1-800-424-9100

National Society to Prevent Blindness
500 E. Remington Road
Schaumburg, IL 60173
(847) 843-2020
1-800-221-3004
1-800-331-2020

Opticians Association of America
10341 Democracy Lane
Fairfax, VA 22030
(703) 691-8355
Fax (703) 691-3929

Volunteer Opportunities
Corporation for National Service
1201 New York Avenue N.W.
Washington, DC 20525-0002
(202) 606-5000

National Federation of Interfaith
Volunteer Caregivers
368 Broadway, Suite 103
Kingston, NY 12401
(914) 331-1358

Retired and Senior Volunteer Program
(RSVP)
National Senior Service Corps Hotline
1-800-424-8867

Volunteers of America, Inc.
110 S. Union Street
Alexandria, VA 22314
1-800-899-0089

Women's Services
American College of Obstetricians
and Gynecologists
409 12th Street S.W.
Washington, DC 20024-2188
(202) 863-2518
1-800-673-8444

Hysterectomy Educational Resources and
Services Foundation
422 Bryn Mawr Avenue
Bala Cynwyd, PA 19004
(610) 667-7757
FAX (610) 667-8096

Meeting the Special Concerns of
Hispanic Older Women
National Hispanic Council on Aging
2713 Ontario Road N.W.
Washington, DC 20009
(202) 265-1288
Fax (202) 745-2522

National Women's Health Network
514 10th Street N.W., Suite 400
Washington, DC 20004
(202) 347-1140
Fax (202) 347-1168

State Area Agencies on Aging and Ombudsman Offices

These addresses and telephone numbers are subject to change. For updated information, you may need to visit the Administration on Aging (AOA) web site: http://www.aca.dhhs.gov/aoa/pages/ltcomb.html (long-term care ombudsman) or http://www.aoa.dhhs.gov/aoa/pages/state.html (Area Agencies on Aging).

	Long-Term Care Ombudsman	State Area Agency on Aging
Alabama	State LTC Ombudsman Alabama Commission on Aging 770 Washington Avenue RSA Plaza, Suite 470 Montgomery, AL 36130 (334) 242-5743 fax (334) 242-5594	Alabama Commission on Aging 770 Washington Avenue RSA Plaza, Suite 470 Montgomery, AL 36130 (334) 242-5743 fax (334) 242-5594
Alaska	Older Alaskans Commission State LTC Ombudsman Office 3601 C Street, Suite 260 Anchorage, AK 99503-5209 (907) 563-6393 fax (907) 561-3862	Alaska Commission on Aging Division of Senior Services Department of Administration P.O. Box 110209 Juneau, AK 99811-0209 (907) 465-3250 fax (907) 465-4716
Arizona	State LTC Ombudsman Aging and Adult Administration 1789 W. Jefferson, 950A Phoenix, AZ 85007 (602) 542-4446 fax (602) 542-6575	Aging and Adult Administration Department of Economic Security 1789 W. Jefferson, #950A Phoenix, AZ 85007 (602) 542-4446 fax (602) 542-6575
Arkansas	Division of Aging and Adult Services State LTC Ombudsman Office P.O. Box 1437 Donaghey Plaza South, Slot 1412 Little Rock, AR 72203-1437 (501) 682-2441 fax (501) 682-8155	Division of Aging and Adult Services Arkansas Department of Human Services P.O. Box 1437, Slot 1412 Little Rock, AR 72203-1437 (501) 682-2441 fax (501) 682-8155

	Long-Term Care Ombudsman	State Area Agency on Aging
California	State LTC Ombudsman California Department of Aging 1600 K Street Sacramento, CA 95814 (916) 323-6681 fax (916) 327-3661	California Department of Aging 1600 K Street Sacramento, CA 95814 (916) 322-5290 fax (916) 324-1903
Colorado	State LTC Ombudsman The Legal Center 455 Sherman Street, Suite 130 Denver, CO 80203-4403 (303) 722-0300 fax (303) 722-0720	Aging and Adult Services Department of Human Services 110 16th Street, Suite 200 Denver, CO 80202-5202 (303) 620-4191 fax (303) 620-4189
Connecticut	State LTC Ombudsman Connecticut Department on Aging Department of Social Services 25 Sigourney Street, 10th Floor Hartford, CT 06106-5033 (860) 424-5200 fax (860) 424-4966	Division of Elderly Services 25 Sigourney Street, 10th Floor Hartford, CT 06106-5033 (860) 424-5277 fax (860) 424-4966
Delaware	State LTC Ombudsman Department of Health and Social Services Division of Services for the Aging and Disabled New Castle County 256 Chapman Road Oxford Building, Suite 200 Newark, DE 19702 (302) 453-3820 fax (302) 453-3836	Delaware Department of Health and Social Services Division of Services for Aging and Adults with Physical Disabilities 1901 N. DuPont Highway, Second Floor Annex New Castle, DE 19720 (302) 577-4791 fax (302) 577-4793
District of Columbia	AARP—Legal Counsel for the Elderly State LTC Ombudsman Office 601 E Street N.W., 4th Floor, Building A Washington, DC 20049 (202) 662-4933 fax (202) 434-6464	District of Columbia Office on Aging 441 Fourth Street N.W. Suite 900 South Washington, DC 20001 (202) 724-5626 fax (202) 724-4979

	Long-Term Care Ombudsman	State Area Agency on Aging
Florida	State LTC Ombudsman Council Carlton Building, Office of the Governor 600 South Calhoun Street, Room 270 Tallahassee, FL 32301-0001 (850) 488-6190 fax (850) 488-5657	Department of Elder Affairs Building B 4040 Esplanade Way, Suite 152 Tallahassee, FL 32399-7000 (850) 414-2000 fax (850) 414-2004
Georgia	State LTC Ombudsman Division of Aging Services Two Peachtree Street N.W., 18th Floor Suite 36-385 Atlanta, GA 30303-3176 (404) 657-5319 fax (404) 657-5285	Division of Aging Services Department of Human Resources Two Peachtree Street N.W. 18th Floor Atlanta, GA 30303 (404) 657-5258 fax (404) 657-5285
Hawaii	State LTC Ombudsman Office of the Governor Hawaii Executive Office on Aging 250 S. Hotel Street, Room 109 Honolulu, HI 96813 (808) 586-0100 fax (808) 586-0185	Hawaii Executive Office on Aging 250 S. Hotel Street, Room 109 Honolulu, HI 96813 (808) 586-0100 fax (808) 586-0185
Idaho	State LTC Ombudsman Idaho Commission on Aging P.O. 3380 Americana Terrace, Suite 120 Boise, ID 83706 (208) 334-3833 fax (208) 334-3033	Idaho Commission on Aging P.O. 3380 Americana Terrace, Suite 120 Boise, ID 83706 (208) 334-3833 fax (208) 334-3033
Illinois	State LTC Ombudsman Illinois Department on Aging 421 E. Capitol Avenue, Suite 100 Springfield, IL 62701-1789 (217) 785-3143 fax (217) 785-4477	Illinois Department on Aging 421 E. Capitol Avenue, Suite 100 Springfield, IL 62701-1789 (217) 785-2870 Chicago office: (312) 814-2630 fax (217) 785-4477

	Long-Term Care Ombudsman	**State Area Agency on Aging**
Indiana	State LTC Ombudsman Division of Disability, Aging and Rehabilitation Services MS 21 P.O. Box 7083-W454 402 W. Washington Street, #W454 Indianapolis, IN 46207-7083 (317) 232-7134 fax (317) 232-7867	Bureau of Aging and In-Home Services Division of Disability, Aging and Rehabilitation Services Family and Social Services Administration MS 21 402 W. Washington Street, #W454 Indianapolis, IN 46207-7083 (317) 232-7020 fax (317) 232-7867
Iowa	State LTC Ombudsman Iowa Department of Elder Affairs Clemens Building 200 Tenth Street, 3rd Floor Des Moines, IA 50309-3609 (515) 281-4656 fax (515) 281-4036	Iowa Department of Elder Affairs Clemens Building 200 Tenth Street, 3rd Floor Des Moines, IA 50309-3609 (515) 281-5187 fax (515) 281-4036
Kansas	State LTC Ombudsman Department on Aging New England Building 503 S. Kansas Topeka, KS 66603-3404 (913) 296-6539 fax (913) 296-0256	Department on Aging New England Building 503 S. Kansas Topeka, KS 66603-3404 (913) 296-4986 fax (913) 296-0256
Kentucky	Kentucky Division of Aging Services State LTC Ombudsman Office 275 E. Main Street, 5th Floor West Frankfort, KY 40602 (502) 564-6930 fax (502) 564-4595	Kentucky Division of Aging Services Cabinet for Human Resources 275 E. Main Street, 6th Floor West Frankfort, KY 40621 (502) 564-6930 fax (502) 564-4595
Louisiana	Governor's Office of Elderly Affairs State LTC Ombudsman Office 412 N. Fourth Street, 3rd Floor Baton Rouge, LA 70802 (504) 342-7100 fax (504) 342-7133	Governor's Office of Elderly Affairs P.O. Box 80374 412 N. Fourth Street, 3rd Floor Baton Rouge, LA 70802 (504) 342-7100 fax (504) 342-7133

	Long-Term Care Ombudsman	**State Area Agency on Aging**
Maine	State LTC Ombudsman Program 21 Bangor Street P.O. Box 126 Augusta, ME 04332-0126 (207) 621-1079 fax (207) 621-0509	Bureau of Elder and Adult Services Department of Human Services 200 Main Street Lewiston, ME 04240 (207) 795-4448 fax (207) 624-5361
Maryland	State LTC Ombudsman Maryland Office on Aging 301 W. Preston Street, Room 1004 Baltimore, MD 21201 (410) 767-1074 fax (410) 333-7943	Maryland Office on Aging State Office Building 301 W. Preston Street, Room 1004 Baltimore, MD 21201-2374 (410) 767-1100 fax (410) 333-7943
Massachusetts	State LTC Ombudsman Massachusetts Executive Office of Elder Affairs One Ashburton Place, 5th Floor Boston, MA 02108-1518 (617) 727-7750 fax (617) 727-9368	Massachusetts Executive Office of Elder Affairs One Ashburton Place, 5th Floor Boston, MA 02108 (617) 727-7750 fax (617) 727-6944
Michigan	Citizens for Better Care State LTC Ombudsman Office 416 N. Homer Street Alpha Building, Suite 101 Lansing, MI 48912-4700 (517) 336-6753 fax (517) 336-7718	Office of Services to the Aging P.O. Box 30676 Lansing, MI 48909-8176 (517) 373-8230 fax (517) 373-4092
Minnesota	Office of Ombudsman 85 E. 7th Place, Suite 280 St. Paul, MN 55101 (651) 296-0382 fax (651) 297-5654	Minnesota Board on Aging 444 Lafayette Road St. Paul, MN 55155-3843 (651) 296-2770 fax (651) 297-7855

	Long-Term Care Ombudsman	**State Area Agency on Aging**
Mississippi	State LTC Ombudsman Division of Aging and Adult Services 750 N. State Street Jackson, MS 39202 (601) 359-4929 fax (601) 359-4970	Division of Aging and Adult Services 750 N. State Street Jackson, MS 39202 (601) 359-4925 fax (601) 359-4370
Missouri	State LTC Ombudsman Missouri Division of Aging Department of Social Services P.O. Box 1337 Jefferson City, MO 65102-1337 (573) 526-0727 fax (573) 751-8687	Missouri Division of Aging Department of Social Services P.O. Box 1337 Jefferson City, MO 65102-1337 (573) 751-3082 fax (573) 751-8687
Montana	State LTC Ombudsman Senior and Long-Term Care Division Department of Public Health and Human Services P.O. Box 4210 Helena, MT 59604 (406) 444-4077 fax (406) 444-7743	Senior and Long-Term Care Division Department of Public Health and Human Services P.O. Box 4210 Helena, MT 59604 (406) 444-4077 fax (406) 444-7743
Nebraska	State LTC Ombudsman Department of Health and Human Services 301 Centennial Mall South P.O. Box 95044 Lincoln, NE 68509-5044 (402) 471-2306 fax (402) 471-4619	Department of Health and Human Services Division on Aging 301 Centennial Mall South P.O. Box 95044 Lincoln, NE 68509-5044 (402) 471-2307 fax (402) 471-4619
Nevada	State LTC Ombudsman Compliance Investigator Department of Human Resources 340 N. 11th Street, Suite 203 Las Vegas, NV 89101 (702) 486-3545 fax (702) 486-3572	Nevada Division for Aging Services Department of Human Resources State Mail Room Complex 340 N. 11th Street, Suite 203 Las Vegas, NV 89101 (702) 486-3545 fax (702) 486-3572

	Long-Term Care Ombudsman	State Area Agency on Aging
New Hampshire	New Hampshire Long-Term Care Ombudsman Program Six Hazen Drive Concord, NH 03301-6505 (603) 271-4375 1-800-443-5640 (in-state only) fax (603) 271-4771	Division of Elderly and Adult Services State Office Park South 115 Pleasant St., Annex Building One Concord, NH 03301-3843 (603) 271-4680 fax (603) 271-4643
New Jersey	Ombudsman Office for Institute for the Elderly 101 S. Broad Street, 6th Floor Trenton, NJ 08625-0808 1-800-792-8820	Department of Health and Senior Services Division of Senior Affairs 101 S. Broad Street, CN 807 Trenton, NJ 08625-0807 (609) 292-2121 1-800-792-8820
New Mexico	State Agency on Aging State LTC Ombudsman Office 228 E. Palace Avenue, Suite A Santa Fe, NM 87501 (505) 827-7663 fax (505) 827-7649	State Agency on Aging La Villa Rivera Building, 4th Floor 228 East Palace Avenue Santa Fe, NM 87501 (505) 827-7640 fax (505) 827-7649
New York	State LTC Ombudsman New York State Office for the Aging Two Empire State Plaza Albany, NY 12223 (518) 474-0108 fax (518) 474-0608	New York State Office for the Aging Two Empire State Plaza Albany, NY 12223 (518) 474-5731 1-800-342-9871 (in-state only) fax (518) 474-0608
North Carolina	State LTC Ombudsman Division of Aging CB 29531 693 Palmer Drive Raleigh, NC 27626-0531 (919) 733-3983 fax (919) 733-0443	Division of Aging CB 29531 693 Palmer Drive Raleigh, NC 27626-0531 (919) 733-3983 fax (919) 733-0443

	Long-Term Care Ombudsman	**State Area Agency on Aging**
North Dakota	State LTC Ombudsman Department of Human Resources Aging Services Division 600 S. 2nd Street, Suite 1C Bismarck, ND 58504 (701) 328-8910 fax (701) 221-5466	Department of Human Services Aging Services Division 600 S. 2nd Street, Suite 1C Bismarck, ND 58504 (701) 328-8910 fax (701) 328-8989
Ohio	State LTC Ombudsman Ohio Department of Aging 50 W. Broad Street, 9th Floor Columbus, OH 43215-5928 (614) 466-7922 fax (614) 466-5741	Ohio Department of Aging 50 West Broad Street, 9th Floor Columbus, OH 43215-5928 (614) 466-5500 fax (614) 466-5741
Oklahoma	State LTC Ombudsman Oklahoma Department of Human Services Aging Services Division 312 N.E. 28th Street Oklahoma City, OK 73105 (405) 521-6734 fax (405) 521-2086	Services for the Aging Oklahoma Department of Human Services P.O. Box 25352 312 N.E. 28th Street Oklahoma City, OK 73105 (405) 521-2281 (405) 521-2327 fax (405) 521-2086
Oregon	Office of the LTC Ombudsman 3855 Wolverine N.E., Suite 6 Salem, OR 97310 (503) 378-6533 fax (503) 373-0852	Senior and Disabled Services Division 500 Summer Street N.E., 2nd Floor Salem, OR 97310-1015 (503) 945-5811 fax 373-7823
Pennsylvania	Pennsylvania Department of Aging LTC Ombudsman Program 555 Walnut Street, 5th Floor Harrisburg, PA 17101-2301 (717) 783-7247 fax (717) 772-3382	Pennsylvania Department of Aging Commonwealth of Pennsylvania 555 Walnut Street, 5th Floor Harrisburg, PA 17101-2301 (717) 783-1550 fax (717) 772-3382

	Long-Term Care Ombudsman	State Area Agency on Aging
Puerto Rico	State LTC Ombudsman Governor's Office of Elderly Affairs CB 50063 Old San Juan Station San Juan, PR 00902 (787) 725-1515 fax (787) 721-6510	Commonwealth of Puerto Rico Governor's Office of Elderly Affairs CB 50063 Old San Juan Station San Juan, PR 00902 (787) 721-5710 (787) 721-4560 (787) 721-6121 fax (787) 721-6510
Rhode Island	State LTC Ombudsman Department of Elderly Affairs 160 Pine Street Providence, RI 02903-3708 (401) 222-2858 fax (401) 277-2130	Department of Elderly Affairs 160 Pine Street Providence, RI 02903-3708 (401) 222-2858 fax (401) 277-1490
South Carolina	State LTC Ombudsman Division on Aging 202 Arbor Lake Drive, Suite 301 Columbia, SC 29223-4535 (803) 737-7500 fax (803) 737-7501	South Carolina Commission on Aging 400 Arbor Lake Drive, Suite B-500 Columbia, SC 29223 (803) 735-0210 fax (803) 786-7752
South Dakota	State LTC Ombudsman Office of Adult Services and Aging Department of Social Services 700 Governors Drive Pierre, SD 57501-2291 (605) 773-3656 fax (605) 773-6834	Office of Adult Services and Aging Richard F. Kneip Building 700 Governors Drive Pierre, SD 57501-2291 (605) 773-3656 fax (605) 773-6834
Tennessee	State LTC Ombudsman Tennessee Commission on Aging Andrew Jackson Building, 9th Floor 500 Deaderick Street Nashville, TN 37243-0860 (615) 741-2056 fax (615) 741-3309	Commission on Aging Andrew Jackson Building, 9th Floor 500 Deaderick Street Nashville, TN 37243-0860 (615) 741-2056 fax (615) 741-3309

	Long-Term Care Ombudsman	**State Area Agency on Aging**
Texas	State LTC Ombudsman Office Texas Department on Aging 4900 N. Lamar Boulevard Austin, TX 78751-2316 (512) 424-6840 fax (512) 424-6890	Texas Department on Aging 4900 North Lamar, 4th Floor Austin, TX 78751 (512) 424-6840 fax (512) 424-6890
Utah	State LTC Ombudsman Department of Human Services Division of Aging and Adult Services 120 N. 200 West, Suite 325 Salt Lake City, UT 84102 (801) 538-3910 fax (801) 538-4395	Department of Human Services Division of Aging and Adult Services 120 N. 200 West, Suite 325 Salt Lake City, UT 84102 (801) 538-3910 fax (801) 538-4395
Vermont	State LTC Ombudsman Vermont Legal Aid 264 N. Winooski P.O. Box 1367 Burlington, VT 05402 (802) 863-5620 fax (802) 863-7152	Vermont Department of Aging and Disabilities Waterbury Complex 103 S. Main Street Waterbury, VT 05676 (802) 241-2400 fax (802) 241-2325
Virginia	State LTC Ombudsman Program Virginia Association of Area Agencies on Aging 530 E. Main Street, Suite 428 Richmond, VA 23219-2327 (804) 644-2923 fax (804) 644-5640	Virginia Department for the Aging 1600 Forest Avenue, Suite 102 Richmond, VA 23229 (804) 662-9333 fax (804) 662-9354
Washington	South King County Multi-Service Center State LTC Ombudsman Office 1200 S. 336th Street Federal Way, WA 98003-7452 (206) 838-6810 fax (206) 874-7831	Aging and Adult Services Administration Department of Social and Health Services P.O. Box 45050 Olympia, WA 98504-5050 (360) 586-8753 fax (360) 902-7848

	Long-Term Care Ombudsman	**State Area Agency on Aging**
West Virginia	DHHR Specialist West Virginia Commission on Aging State LTC Ombudsman Office 1900 Kanawha Boulevard East Holly Grove, Building 10 Charleston, WV 25305-0160 (304) 558-3317 fax (304) 558-0004	Commission on Aging 1900 Kanawha Boulevard East Holly Grove, Building 10 Charleston, WV 25305-0160 (304) 558-3317 fax (304) 558-0004
Wisconsin	State LTC Ombudsman Board on Aging and Long-Term Care 214 N. Hamilton Street Madison, WI 53703-2118 (608) 266-8944 fax (608) 261-6570	Bureau of Aging and Long-Term Care Resources Department of Health and Family Services 217 S. Hamilton Street, Suite 300 Madison, WI 53703 (608) 266-2536 fax (608) 267-3203
Wyoming	State LTC Ombudsman Wyoming Senior Citizens, Inc. 756 Gilchrist P.O. Box 94 Wheatland, WY 82201 (307) 322-5553 fax (307) 322-3283	Division on Aging Department of Health 139 Hathaway Building Cheyenne, WY 82002-0480 (307) 777-7986 fax (307) 777-5340
Guam		Division of Senior Citizens Department of Public Health and Social Services P.O. Box 2816 Agana, Guam 96910 (671) 632-4141 fax (671) 637-0333

	Long-Term Care Ombudsman	**State Area Agency on Aging**
North Mariana Islands		Office on Aging Department of Community and Cultural Affairs Civic Center Commonwealth of the North Mariana Islands Saipan, MP 96950 (671) 734-4361 fax (671) 477-2930
Palau		Republic of Palau Agency on Aging Republic of Palau Koror, PW 96940 (680) 488-2736 fax (680) 488-1662 fax (680) 488-1597
American Samoa		Territorial Administration on Aging Government of American Samoa Pago Pago, American Samoa 96799 (684) 633-2207 fax (684) 633-2533 fax (684) 633-7723
Virgin Islands		Senior Citizen Affairs Virgin Islands Department of Human Services 19 Estate Diamond Fredericksted St. Croix, VI 00840 (809) 772-4950 ext. 46 fax (809) 692-2062

Home Healthcare Hotlines

If you have a problem or complaint about a home healthcare agency or service, report the problem to your state home healthcare hotline. This network was originally set up to gather information about Medicare-certified home healthcare agencies. However, in many states, these offices also address broader health-care issues. They will generally not make referrals, but they may answer questions or tell you if a particular agency has been the subject of complaints.

Alabama
1-800-225-9770

Alaska
1-907-563-0037

Arizona
1-800-221-9968

Arkansas
1-800-223-0340

California
- Berkeley
 1-800-554-0352
- Chico
 1-800-554-0350
- Daly City
 1-800-554-0353
- Fresno
 1-800-554-0351
- Los Angeles
 1-800-228-1019
- Orange County
 1-800-228-5234
- Sacramento
 1-800-554-0354
- San Bernadino
 1-800-344-2896

- San Diego
 1-800-824-0613
- San Jose
 1-800-554-0348
- Santa Rosa
 1-800-554-0349
- Ventura
 1-800-547-8267

Colorado
1-800-842-8826

Connecticut
1-800-828-9769

Delaware
1-800-942-7373

District of Columbia
1-202-727-7873

Florida
1-800-962-6014

Georgia
1-800-326-0291

Hawaii
1-800-762-5949

Idaho
1-800-345-1453

Illinois
1-800-252-4343

Indiana
1-800-227-6334

Iowa
1-800-281-4920

Kansas
1-800-842-0078

Kentucky
1-800-635-6290

Louisiana
1-800-327-3419

Maine
1-800-621-8222

Maryland
1-800-492-6005

Massachusetts
1-800-462-5540

Michigan
1-800-882-6006

Minnesota
1-800-369-7994

Mississippi
1-800-227-7308

Missouri
1-800-877-6485

Montana
1-800-762-4618

Nebraska
1-800-245-5832

Nevada
1-800-225-3414

New Hampshire
1-800-621-6232

New Jersey
1-800-792-9770

New Mexico
1-800-752-8649

New York
1-800-628-5972

North Carolina
1-800-624-3004

North Dakota
1-800-545-8256

Ohio
1-800-342-0553

Oklahoma
1-800-234-7258

Oregon
1-800-542-5186

Pennsylvania
1-800-692-7254

Puerto Rico
1-809-721-5710

Rhode Island
1-800-277-2788

South Carolina
1-800-922-6735

South Dakota
1-800-592-1861

Tennessee
1-800-541-7367

Texas
1-800-228-1570

Utah
1-800-999-7339

Vermont
1-800-564-1612

Virginia
1-800-955-1819

Virgin Islands
1-809-774-2991

Washington
1-800-633-6828

West Virginia
1-800-442-2888

Wisconsin
1-800-642-6552

Wyoming
1-800-548-1367

Internet Sites

The following is a list of helpful Internet resources. Most of these sites also have excellent links to other web sites with related information.

Organizations

Administration on Aging's Directory of Web Sites on Aging
http://www.aoa.dhhs.gov/aoa/webres/craig.htm

Administration on Aging's Family Caregiving Options
http://www.aoa.dhhs.gov/aoa/webres/family-G.htm

Advice and Consent
http://www.adviceconsent.com

Age of Reason
http://www.ageofreason.com

Aging with Dignity
http://www.agingwithdignity.org

Alzheimer's Association
http://www.alz.org

American Association of Homes and Services for the Aging
http://www.spry.org

American Association of Retired Persons
http://www.aarp.org

American Medical Association
http://www.ama-assn.org

American Psychiatric Association
http://www.psych.org

American Red Cross
http://www.crossnet.org

B'nai B'rith
http://seniors@bnaibrith.org

Bureau of Elder and Adult Services Resource Directory
http://www.state.me.us/beas/resource.htm

255

Caregiver Network Inc.
http://www.caregiver.on.ca

Caregiver Resources
http://www.ianet.org/multiuse.care_giv.htm

Caregiver Survivor Resources
http://www.caregiver911.com

The Caregiver's Handbook
http://www.acsu.buffalo.edu/~drstall/hndbk0.html

Caregiving Online
http://www.caregiving.com

Catholic Charities USA
http://ccsj.org/senior.html

Choice In Dying, Inc.
http://www.choices.org

Community Transportation Association of America
http://www.ctaa.org

Consumer Information Center
http://www.pueblo.gsa.gov

Council of Better Business Bureaus, Inc.
http://www.bbb.org

Eldercare Navigator
http://www.mindspring.com

Eldercare Web
http://www.elderweb.com

Elderhostel
http://www.elderhostel.com

Elderlinks
http://www.ink.org/public/keln/keln_links.html

Federal Trade Commission
http://www.ftc.gov

Fifty Plus.Net
http://www.fifty-plus.net

GoldenAge.Net
http://www.elo.mediasrv.swt.edu/goldenage/script.htm

Guide to Retirement Living
http://www.retirement-living.com

Healthcare Financing Administration (Medicare and Medicaid)
http://www.hcfa.gov

Hospice Hands
http://www.hospice-cares.com

Insurance Information Institute
http://www.iii.org

Joint Commission on Accreditation of Healthcare Organizations
http://www.jcaho.org

This List is 100% Solid Gold
http://pw2.netcom.com/~lehdoll/solidGOLD.html

Long-Term Care
http://www.hrfn.net/~ltcare/ltc.htm

My Virtual Reference Desk—Seniors Online
http://www.refdesk.com/seniors.html

National Aging Information Center
http://www.ageinfo.org

National Association for Home Care
http://www.nahc.org

National Committee for Quality Assurance
http://www.ncqa.org

National Fraud Information Center
http://www.fraud.org

National Hospice Organization
http://www.nho.org

National Institutes of Health
http://www.nih.gov

Nursing Home INFO
http://www.nursinghomeinfo.com

Nursing Home Information Site
http://members.tripod.com/~volfangary/index.html

SeniorCom
http://www.senior.com

Senior Information Network
http://www.senior-inet.com

Senior Law
http://www.seniorlaw.com

Senior Net
http://www.seniornet.org

Senior Options
http://www.senioroptions.com

Social Security Administration
http://www.ssa.gov

Third Age
http://www.thirdage.com

U.S. Department of Health and Human Services
http://www.os.dhhs.gov

U.S. Department of Housing and Urban Development
http://www.hud.gov

General Directory Assistance

Yahoo People Search
http://people.yahoo.com

Switchboard
http://www.switchboard.com

Search Engines

Yahoo
http://www.yahoo.com/Health/Geriatrics_and_Aging

AltaVista
http://altavista.looksmart.com/r?lm&izf&e53796